Pocket Guide to Perioperative and Critical Care Echocardiography

D1354486

Pocket Guide to Perioperative and Critical Care Echocardiography

Colin Royse MBBS, MD, FANZCA
Course Co-director of the Postgraduate Diploma of
Perioperative and Critical Care Echocardiography,
The University of Melbourne
Co-Head of the Human Cardiovascular Research
Laboratory, Department of Pharmacology, The
University of Melbourne

Garry Donnan MBBS, FANZCA, PTEeXAM
Staff Anaesthetist, Royal Melbourne Hospital

Alistair Royse MBBS, MD, FRACS
Course Co-director of the Postgraduate Diploma of
Perioperative and Critical Care Echocardiography,
The University of Melbourne

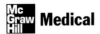

Medical

National Library of Australia Cataloguing-in-Publication data:

Royse, Colin.
McGraw-Hill's pocket guide to perioperative and critical care echocardiography.

Bibliography.
Includes index.
ISBN 0 074 71611 5.

1. Echocardiography. 2. Heart – Diseases – Diagnosis. I. Donnan, Garry. II. Royse, Alistair. III. Title. IV. Title : Pocket guide to preoperative and critical care echocardiography.

616. 1207543

Published in Australia by
McGraw-Hill Australia Pty Ltd
Level 2, 82 Waterloo Road, North Ryde NSW 2113
Publisher: Nicole Meehan
Production Editor: Sybil Kesteven
Editor: Kerry Brown
Proofreader: Tim Learner
Indexer: Glenda Browne
Designer (cover and interior): Lara Scott, Unhinged Productions
Illustrator: Alan Laver, Shelly Communications
CD development and design: FutureTrain
Typeset in 8.5/11pt Sabon by Midland Typesetters, Australia
Printed on 80 gsm matt art by 1010 Printing International Ltd, China

The McGraw·Hill Companies

Foreword

The use of ultrasound is rapidly emerging as an integral part of the practice of perioperative and critical care medicine. Development of the available ultrasound modalities has lead to an expanded role for clinicians in anaesthesia, critical care and emergency medicine.

Transoesophageal echocardiography is extremely useful for the assessment of patients with inexplicable haemodynamic disturbances, and has important applications in cardiac and vascular surgery, as well as in the intensive care unit. The increasing importance of surface ultrasound as a tool for both vascular imaging and neural blockade is recognised. Point-of-care ultrasound also improves intervention efficacy and enhances patient safety. Focused assessment with sonography for trauma has already largely superseded abdominal peritoneal lavage in the emergency department, and other point-of-care uses are rapidly evolving.

The Royal Melbourne Hospital is a tertiary referral university hospital at which ultrasound is used extensively. The contributors are all experienced ultrasound practitioners and teachers, and the editors' expertise covers cardiac surgery, perioperative medicine and academic anaesthesia through their affiliation with The University of Melbourne.

This book is excellent for the novice learning about ultrasound and echocardiography, and also provides a comprehensive overview of perioperative and critical care ultrasound for more experienced clinicians. There is an emphasis on the development of a directed examination and understanding the technology's limitations. The accompanying compact disc supports the text and illustrations.

I believe this book will become an essential reference for all clinicians interested in both echocardiography and the other uses of medical ultrasound.

Daryl Williams FANZCA
Director
Department of Anaesthesia and Pain Management
Royal Melbourne Hospital

Contents

Foreword   v
List of contributors   xi
Note from the editors   xiii
Acknowledgments   xiv

Chapter 1 Ultrasound in perioperative and critical care clinical practice   1
Development of medical ultrasound imaging   1
Uses of perioperative and critical care echocardiography   2
Transoesophageal versus transthoracic echocardiography   4
Uses of point-of-care ultrasound   6
Future developments   8

Chapter 2 Understanding the echocardiography machine   9
Basic ultrasound physics   9
Echocardiography equipment   11
Imaging modes   15
Doppler effect and Doppler imaging modes   15
Limitations in echocardiography   18

Chapter 3 Obtaining the best ultrasound image   20
Factors affecting the ultrasound image   20
Instrument layout and settings   21
Room configuration   29
Artefacts and pitfalls   30

Chapter 4 Core anatomy for echocardiography   38
Overview of thoracic anatomy   38
Overview of cardiac anatomy   41
Variations in individual anatomy and implications for echocardiography   46
Echocardiography 'blind spots'   47

Chapter 5 Standard transoesophageal echocardiography examination   49
Care of the probe   49
The standard examination   50

**Chapter 6 Standard transthoracic echocardiography
    examination**   63
    Positioning the patient   63
    The basic windows   64
    The standard examination   69

Chapter 7 Introduction to Doppler imaging and equations   73
    Understanding Doppler imaging   73
    The standard Doppler examination   84
    Estimating right atrial pressure   88
    Calculating cardiac output and area of valves   88
    Summary of the equations   90

Chapter 8 Assessing the basic haemodynamic state   93
    The basic haemodynamic states   93
    The basic haemodynamic assessment   94
    Value of haemodynamic diagnosis in patient management   104

Chapter 9 Problems with ventricles   110
    Global ventricular function   110
    Ischaemic heart disease   112
    Cardiomyopathies   113
    Regional wall motion abnormalities   116
    Assessing diastolic function   118
    Cardiac masses and locating a potential cardiac source
        of embolus   125

Chapter 10 Problems with valves   131
    Aortic valve   131
    Mitral valve   137
    Tricuspid valve   143
    Pulmonary valve   145
    Evaluation of valvular stenosis   147
    Evaluation of valvular regurgitation   149
    Evaluation of prosthetic valves   150
    Endocarditis   154

Chapter 11 Problems with great vessels 156
   Evaluation of the great vessels 156
   Aortic dissection in the emergency department 159
   Repair of aortic dissection or aneurysm 160
   Other aortic pathology 161
   Assessment of atheroma with epiaortic ultrasound 162
   Assessment of pulmonary embolism 163

Chapter 12 Problems with pericardium and pleura 164
   Assessment of pericardial and pleural disease 164
   Pericardial effusion 166
   Pericardial tamponade 169
   Limitations in diagnosing pericardial pathology 176

Chapter 13 Ultrasound-guided regional anaesthesia 177
   Development of ultrasound-guided regional anaesthesia 177
   Ultrasonography of nerves 178
   The brachial plexus 181
   The lumbosacral plexus 186
   Peripheral nerves 189

Chapter 14 Ultrasound-guided vascular access 190
   Development of ultrasound-guided vascular access 190
   Equipment requirements 191
   Cannulation techniques 192
   Cannulation of specific vessels 195
   How to differentiate arteries from veins 199

Chapter 15 Education and training 200
   Getting started in ultrasound 200
   Standards 202
   Further educational opportunities 202

References and further reading 203
Glossary 207
Index 212

List of contributors

David Andrews MBBS, FANZCA, PTEeXAM
Staff Anaesthetist, Royal Melbourne Hospital
Clinical interests include cardiac anaesthesia, transoesophageal
  echocardiography and myocardial protection during
  cardiopulmonary bypass

Peter Dawson MBBS, FANZCA, PTEeXAM
Visiting Specialist Anaesthetist, Royal Melbourne Hospital

Garry Donnan MBBS, FANZCA, PTEeXAM
Staff Anaesthetist, Royal Melbourne Hospital
Clinical interests include cardiac anaesthesia, echocardiography,
  medical perfusion and intradermal testing for suspected
  anaphylaxis

John Faris DAvMed, FAFOM, FFOM, FANZCA, BA, PTEeXAM
Specialist Anaesthetist, Sir Charles Gairdner Hospital, Perth, WA
Specialist anaesthetist and occupational physician with interests
  in cardiothoracic anaesthesia and echocardiography, aviation
  medicine and information technology

Robyn Gillies MBBS (Hons), FANZCA, PTEeXAM
Consultant Anaesthetist and Head of Malignant Hyperthermia
  Diagnostic Unit, Department of Anaesthesia and Pain
  Management, Royal Melbourne Hospital
American Board of Echocardiography Certification 2003

Colin Iatrou MBBS, FANZCA, PTEeXAM
Visiting Anaesthetist, Royal Melbourne Hospital
Clinical interests include cardiac anaesthesia, echocardiography
  and medical perfusion

Ruari Orme MBBS, FANZCA, PostGradDipEcho, PTEeXAM
Staff Anaesthetist, Royal Melbourne Hospital
Clinical interests include cardiac anaesthesia, regional anaesthesia
  and analgesia, and first part FANZCA training

Alistair Royse MBBS, MD, FRACS
Course Co-director of the Postgraduate Diploma of Perioperative
  and Critical Care Echocardiography, The University of
  Melbourne
Cardiothoracic surgery and general surgery fellowships
Doctoral thesis on composite arterial coronary artery bypass surgery

Colin Royse MBBS, MD, FANZCA
Course Co-director of the Postgraduate Diploma of Perioperative
  and Critical Care Echocardiography, The University of
  Melbourne
Co-Head of the Human Cardiovascular Research Laboratory,
  Department of Pharmacology, The University of Melbourne
Visiting Anaesthetist, Royal Melbourne Hospital

Reny Segal MBChB, FANZCA, PTEeXAM
Staff Specialist, Department of Anaesthesia and Pain Management,
  Royal Melbourne Hospital

Paul Soeding MBBS, BSc (Hons), FANZCA, PTEeXAM
Consultant Anaesthetist, Department of Anaesthesia and Pain
  Management, Royal Melbourne Hospital
Senior Fellow, Department of Pharmacology, The University of
  Melbourne

Gerard Stainsby MBBS, FANZCA, PTEeXAM
Visiting Specialist Anaesthetist, Royal Melbourne Hospital
Clinical interests include cardiothoracic anaesthesia, transoesophageal
  echocardiography, medical physics and computers

Joan Sutherland MBBS, FRCPC, FANZCA
Staff Anaesthetist, Royal Melbourne Hospital
Clinical interests include cardiac anaesthesia, perioperative
  echocardiography and management of diabetes mellitus

Michael Veltman MBBS, FANZCA, PTEeXAM, ASCeXAM
Staff Specialist, Department of Anaesthesia and Pain Medicine,
  Royal Perth Hospital
Specialist cardiothoracic anaesthetist with an interest in
  perioperative and diagnostic echocardiography

Berthold Weitkamp FANZCA, FRCA, PTEeXAM
Staff Specialist, Department of Anaesthesia and Pain Management,
  Royal Melbourne Hospital

Note from the editors

The aim of this book is to introduce you to the practice of echocardiography and ultrasound. Chapters 1–4 provide background information to help you understand the equipment, relevant indications and core anatomical features used in this form of imaging. Chapters 5 and 6 outline the standard procedure for transoesophageal and transthoracic examinations, and Chapter 7 covers the Doppler examination, including the equations used to quantify echocardiography parameters. Chapters 8–12 describe the echocardiographic findings for specific cardiovascular pathologies and Chapters 13 and 14 give an overview of the applications of surface ultrasound, which is being increasingly used in perioperative medicine (i.e. nerve blocks and vascular access). Finally, Chapter 15 presents suggestions for getting started with ultrasound and for further education in this technique. A list of references is provided for those wishing to delve more into the topic and a glossary gives definitions of specific terms and abbreviations.

How to use this book

The CD icon that appears throughout the text—for example, on page 3—indicates that there is a video clip in the relevant chapter on the mini-CD. You must have QuickTime™ V5 or later installed on your computer to view the videos.

On loading the mini-CD the software will check if your computer has QuickTime installed. If QuickTime is not installed it will ask you if you wish to install it. Select Yes and QuickTime will be automatically installed from a file on the mini-CD. The installation takes about 30 seconds. To play the video clips, load the mini-CD and follow the instructions on screen. (See also the last page of this book.)

Acknowledgments

The editors extend special thanks to all members of the Department of Pharmacology, The University of Melbourne and the Department of Anaesthesia and Pain Management, Royal Melbourne Hospital for their support during preparation of the manuscript.

They also thank Ms Danielle Nicholas, Echocardiography Technologist, Cardiovascular Therapeutics Unit, Department of Pharmacology, The University of Melbourne for her assistance with the diagrams, video files and proofreading, and Mrs Marcelle Wood for administrative support.

The expert assistance provided by McGraw-Hill Australia is gratefully acknowledged.

Colin Royse
Garry Donnan
Alistair Royse

Chapter 1

Ultrasound in perioperative and critical care clinical practice

Robyn Gillies

Learning objectives

1. Understand the multiple roles of ultrasound and echocardiography in the perioperative environment.
2. Understand uses of ultrasound and echocardiography in the critical care and emergency department environments.
3. Understand the contraindications and limitations of ultrasound and echocardiography.

Development of medical ultrasound imaging

Medical use of ultrasound can trace its origins from technology developed from the principles of SONAR (sound navigation and ranging) in the 1800s. One of the first recorded uses of echocardiography was in the early 1950s by Inge Edler and Carl Hertz at the University Hospital in Lund, Sweden. They characterised the movement of the mitral valve in mitral stenosis and correlated this with surgical findings.

The application of continuous wave Doppler measurements in 1963, the development of real-time scanners in 1965 and the use of pulsed Doppler in 1970 increased the potential uses of medical ultrasound, but it was not until 1974 when the first duplex pulsed-Doppler scanner was developed that echocardiography became a more viable diagnostic tool. The duplex scanner (i.e. 2D imaging combined with Doppler signals) enabled placement and visual location of the ultrasound beam, thus obtaining position information for flow measurements. Another significant development was the use of colour Doppler in Japan in the 1980s.

Although diagnostic ultrasound as a radiology and cardiology specialty has been available for many years, it is only recently with the advent of smaller machines and increasing availability of ultrasound, better 'post-production' display of the signals, and improved medical knowledge, that echocardiography and ultrasound have become a vital part of the diagnostic and monitoring armamentarium of the anaesthetist, the emergency physician and the critical care physician.

Increasing use of the modalities brings with it the advantages of rapid assessment and immediate feedback for life-threatening conditions, and echocardiography can be used as an additional haemodynamic and intraoperative monitor. The potential disadvantages of decreased accuracy with untrained operators and limited information obtained from scans performed in the perioperative setting can be overcome with appropriate training and accreditation of operators, and the use of guidelines for imaging examinations.

Uses of perioperative and critical care echocardiography

There is great benefit to be obtained from using echocardiography in the perioperative and critical care environments. Rapidly changing haemodynamics of a patient, or the need to rule out life-threatening conditions in the operating room, ICU or ED, shifts the focus of echocardiography from conventional radiological diagnosis to a limited, usually time constrained, directed examination. Standard views and examinations have been developed for both transthoracic (TTE) and transoesophageal echocardiography (TOE or TEE) and are detailed in Chapters 5 and 6.

Use of TOE

The usefulness of TOE in guiding clinical diagnosis and patient management has been studied and recommendations for the use of perioperative TOE have been developed. There is little controversy about using TOE in life-threatening emergencies and it has become routine practice for cardiac surgery in many centres worldwide. It is being increasingly used in trauma practice, not only to identify the patient's haemodynamic state, but also structural damage to the heart and aorta.

The use of ultrasound is potentially unlimited; however, although surface ultrasound is safe, TOE is an invasive procedure with a risk of oesophageal perforation, and despite that risk being low, it is a complication that can prove fatal. Therefore, TOE should not be used without justifiable indications for its use. It is important to note that the use of echocardiography has changed considerably since the indications were published in 1996.

Examples of the use of TOE in non-cardiac surgery include cases of trauma, patients with persistent hypotension, known vascular disease, undergoing percutaneous pacemaker/defibrillator lead extraction, or with a history of left heart failure, and it may be used as a guide for intraoperative fluid therapy and the possible use of inotropes and vasodilators during liver and lung transplantation. It has enormous value as an intraoperative monitor of the patient's response to interventions and changes in conditions.

Use of TTE

For many years TTE has been used for the diagnosis of acute and chronic cardiac conditions. Its value to the intensivist is the ability to assess inexplicable haemodynamic disturbances when other tests are unavailable or inappropriate. It can be used for 'snapshot' monitoring of the patient's response to therapy, assessment of left and/or right ventricular systolic function, diagnosis of regional wall motion abnormalities in cases of suspected ischaemia, assessment of valvular function, examination of the pericardium and pulmonary tree, and diagnosis of acute thoracic aortic problems such as dissection.

Critical care physicians who are trained in the use of echocardiography are able to accurately diagnose conditions that require immediate intervention, such as cardiac tamponade, and TTE is specifically used to assess patient response to fluid administration in the ICU setting, with IVC responsiveness as the measured parameter.

The increasing use and greater availability of TTE in the ICU may help decrease the need for invasive cardiac monitoring. Other uses in the ICU include 'point-of-care' which is detailed later.

Transoesophageal versus transthoracic echocardiography

The decision to use TOE or TTE will be mainly dictated by the patient's general condition. Other factors influencing the decision include the relatively invasive nature of TOE and the requirement in some cases for sedation and/or airway intubation for a full TOE examination to be carried out. TTE on the other hand is non-invasive and can be performed in the fully awake patient. Contraindications to TOE (both absolute and relative) will also influence the choice of technique. Another factor to consider is the level of expertise with echocardiography in perioperative practice. The initial use of TOE was for cardiac surgery, which requires a high level of operator expertise, but nowadays it is logical for the novice to start using surface ultrasound applications, such as limited TTE, vascular access or nerve blocks, before progressing to TOE.

Risks of TOE and TTE
The safety of ultrasound in terms of tissue damage is well established, but there are still some important risks, both actual and theoretical, associated with the use of TOE and TEE. The first and foremost risk of any diagnostic modality is misinterpreting the results, leading to incorrect and/or potentially harmful interventions based on this information. Training and the setting of standards for basic TOE and TEE examinations are aimed at minimising this risk, and are essential for the successful and safe use of echocardiography by the intensivist, anaesthetist or emergency physician.

Other risks inherent to the use of TOE include dental trauma (0.1%), oesophageal trauma or perforation (<0.1%), bleeding, aspiration, and dislodgement or displacement of the endotracheal or nasogastric tube. Dysphagia and lip injuries, and reversible tongue staining by the disinfectant, are potential adverse effects. There is also the theoretical risk of transmission of infection in an inadequately cleaned probe.

Limitations and considerations

Both TTE and TOE will be of limited value if the views are inadequate for diagnosis, which can be influenced by body habitus. TTE is more difficult in obese or emphysematous patients, and TOE views from the stomach can be affected by a hiatus hernia or the stomach being full of air.

TTE may be more accurate for assessing the continuous wave Doppler for aortic gradients because the relationship between the oesophagus, trachea and left main bronchus means TOE is unable to provide a view of the origin of most of the aortic arch vessels. However, TOE does give a more accurate (closer) view of smaller cardiac structures and pathology, such as vegetations on valves.

In situations where the anaesthetist is the sole operator the TOE examination may be less than satisfactory because it may be unsafe to do anything more than a limited examination while simultaneously monitoring with other modalities and providing anaesthesia. The increasing use of TOE as an intraoperative monitor requires changes in the number of anaesthesia staff, especially during the operator's learning period.

The interpretation of the ultrasound images is affected by artifacts caused by the physical properties of ultrasound and/or the machine used to propagate the sound waves. The presence of misleading artifacts or misinterpretation of normal structures that leads to misdiagnosis is potentially dangerous in the perioperative setting.

When considering TOE as a monitoring or diagnostic tool, the usefulness of the information that may be obtained must be weighed against the dangers of its use in certain circumstances. It is also important to remember that force should not be used to advance the TOE probe in the oesophagus and that the probe should always be straight when moving it in and out of the oesophagus. The advent of a TOE probe with endoscopic guidance may increase the safety of the procedure.

There are a few absolute contraindications to the use of TOE: a vascular ring, tracheo-oesophageal fistula, oesophageal stricture or obstruction, perforated hollow viscus or active gastrointestinal bleeding. Relative contraindications include oesophageal varices, Barrett's oesophagus, Zenker's diverticulum, oesophageal deformity, previous oesophageal surgery, post radiation therapy of the oesophageal area and severe coagulopathy. The benefits versus risks of TOE should be considered for frail elderly patients, patients with mediastinal disease and those with a previous history of other gastric disorders.

Uses of point-of-care ultrasound

Point-of-care ultrasound (i.e. at the bedside or in the operating room or ED) has become an important clinical tool for critical care physicians, anaesthetists and emergency physicians. The goal is to perform a directed examination rather than full diagnostic testing, with an understanding of the limitations of the particular examination.

Focused assessment with sonography for trauma (FAST)

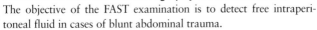

The objective of the FAST examination is to detect free intraperitoneal fluid in cases of blunt abdominal trauma.

Directed ultrasound examination to detect intraperitoneal and pericardial fluid through the use of four standard windows began being developed in the 1970s. Its widespread use in the 1990s, with an increasing number of evidence-based studies, has led to FAST becoming an integral part of the initial trauma examination. Guidelines for the examination and listing of 'inconclusive' findings that require further diagnostic examination (if the patient is stable enough) define its safety and efficacy in the ED. The danger is that FAST may be used to perform a more extensive examination than it is validated for, increasing the possibility of wrong or misleading diagnoses and thus potential harm to the patient.

Imaging of vascular structures

Handheld ultrasound devices that are used to locate vascular structures or determine the presence of venous thrombosis have been available for many years. Static ultrasound without the use of a probe for guidance is of some use, but the recent development of dynamic ultrasound using a sterile sheath over a probe has proved to be even more successful.

In the ICU and ED point-of-care ultrasound is used to define the location of arterial bleeding and thus indicate the area for direct pressure and maximal chance of controlling haemorrhage. Intraoperative epiaortic scanning is used to identify atheroma in the ascending aorta (mid portion of the arch of the aorta where TOE views are obscured by the trachea and left main bronchus) and thus help determine the site of cannulation and cross-clamping of the aorta.

Imaging of nerve bundles

The use of ultrasound to direct nerve block of a major plexus is increasing and may lead to a reduction in complications and increased

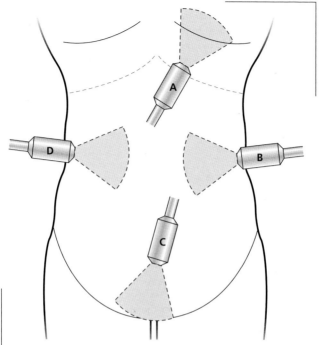

Figure 1.1 The four FAST ultrasound windows.
A: pericardial, B: perisplenic, C: pelvic, D: perihepatic

success rate. Its value is both avoidance of other anatomical structures and location of the correct site for nerve catheters and injection of local anaesthetic. Two procedures that have been well studied are locating the brachial plexus and the femoral nerve, and other areas of study are caudal block and guided sciatic nerve block. The safety of ultrasound-guided nerve blocks will improve with advances in the technology, providing visual input into what is traditionally a non-visual procedure.

Applications in the ICU
Percutaneous tracheostomy: Avoiding vascular structures and identifying aberrant anatomy are two areas where ultrasound can be a useful aid to percutaneous tracheostomy in the ICU.

Ultrasound-guided thoracentesis and pericardiocentesis: Ultrasound can be used to diagnose a pneumothorax. Locating the best area for pleural and pericardial drainage with real-time ultrasound guidance has the potential to decrease morbidity from such procedures. However, using point-of-care ultrasound to drain non-clinically significant effusions is inappropriate.

Urinary retention: Ultrasound has been used for many years to assess urinary retention and it can be also used to guide the placement of suprapubic catheters.

Obstetric applications: Using ultrasound to detect fetal movement and acute placental abnormalities may have application in the critical care environment.

Intraoperative uses: Ultrasound and Doppler have been used during neurosurgical operations to detect residual flow in cerebral aneurysms and to locate tumours. Its use is well established in breast and vascular surgery, gynaecology, urology and intra-abdominal laparoscopic surgery. Recently, the safety of transbronchial biopsies of lung lesions has been improved by the use of ultrasound guidance.

Future developments

As technology advances, smaller, more user-friendly scanners will become available. Better post-production imaging and the use of 3D technology will help to alleviate some of the problems with the interpretation of images in two dimensions. Artefacts will diminish in importance and the scans will be less open to misinterpretation, thus increasing the safety profile of diagnostic ultrasound.

However, it will always be essential for medical graduates to have a basic understanding of the principles and common uses of ultrasound. The development of guidelines for directed examinations, regular reassessment of the evidence for the use of ultrasound in the perioperative, intensive care and emergency settings and the appropriate accreditation of those involved in diagnostic decision-making are vital components in the future of critical care ultrasound.

Chapter 2

Understanding the echocardiography machine

Gerard Stainsby

Learning objectives

1. Understand the function of the components of modern echocardiography machines.
2. Understand the basic physics as it relates to clinical use.
3. Understand the limitations in the use of ultrasound.

Basic ultrasound physics

Sound is a wave of alternating compression and rarefaction that propagates through a physical medium. Frequencies from approximately 20 Hz to 20 kHz can be heard by the human ear. Ultrasound refers to frequencies beyond this range.

Medical ultrasound imaging is the controlled transmission of a beam of sound energy into the body tissues and subsequent detection of the echoes that arise as the beam encounters interfaces within the area of interest. Ultrasound is convenient for imaging because unlike visible light, sound transmits through the body reasonably well, although it has difficulty penetrating bone and air-filled spaces. Unlike X-rays, ultrasound at moderate power levels appears to be harmless to tissues, can be used during pregnancy, and does not inconveniently irradiate nearby staff. The equipment is relatively compact, simple and robust, and the transducer elements can be made very small.

A sound wave has properties, such as frequency, wavelength and amplitude, and is subject to processes such as reflection, refraction, and interference. The propagation speed depends on the physical properties of the medium, and in air is approximately 345 m/s. Water is approximately 800-fold denser than air, and far less compressible, and the resulting speed of sound in water (and thus body tissues) is generally taken to be 1540 m/s. The Doppler effect is important for analysing velocities (see later).

The length λ, frequency f and propagation speed c of a wave are interrelated: $\lambda = c/f$.

Because the desired wavelength for medical ultrasound imaging is less than 1 mm, frequencies in the megahertz range are required. The frequency used is a trade-off between image resolution, which improves with higher frequencies, versus attenuation of the beam (with depth), which worsens as the frequency increases. The posterior cardiac structures lie close to the oesophagus, so TOE is typically able to take advantage of higher frequencies than TTE.

Reflection of sound waves occurs when the wave encounters an interface at which the acoustic impedance changes. The amplitude of the echo arising from an acoustic interface depends on the degree of impedance mismatch. Most tissues share similar acoustic imped- ances, so only a small amount of energy is reflected from these inter- faces and the resultant echoes are very faint. The mismatch between air and the tissues is so great that essentially all ultrasound energy is reflected from this interface—hence the need for a coupling medium (gel) for transthoracic imaging.

The imaging algorithm attributes all echoes to the direction of the last emitted ultrasound beam. The distance from the transducer to the reflecting object is computed from the time interval from the transmission of the ultrasound pulse to the reception of the echo, with the speed of sound in the tissues assumed to be a constant. Each centimetre of depth adds approximately 13 microseconds to the total time.

Range resolution is limited by the spatial pulse length, and so most imaging modes use very short 'pings' (i.e. pulses) that are only a few wavelengths long. A continuously emitted beam does not permit determination of range.

Several processes cause a reduction in the amplitude of the ultrasound beam as it penetrates the tissues. Absorption by the medium (losing the ultrasound energy as heat) depends on the frequency of the beam. The energy that returns to the transducer as echoes is also lost, and a very bright echo is often associated with acoustic shadowing because there is insufficient energy to be reflected back from deeper structures to the transducer.

Although the ultrasound beam emitted by the transducer is reasonably directional in the near field, the inverse-square law applies to the echoes as they arise because interfaces are generally irregular and give rise to scattered reflections. In the far field, divergence of the original beam also reduces its amplitude.

The net result of these processes is that the intensity of echoes, as detected by the transducer, falls off enormously as the distance to the source increases. The electronics of the detector amplifier are designed to suitably increase the gain (ratio of output amplitude to input amplitude) to compensate for this effect. A user-adjustable time gain control (usually a series of horizontally arranged sliders) can fine-tune the gain of the system. The desired result is that the echoes of similar structures give rise to similar screen brightness regardless of their depth.

Ideally, all of the ultrasound energy transmitted into the tissues goes in the direction desired for imaging. In practice, some energy is lost in other directions (side-lobes). A bright reflector struck by a side-lobe will generate echoes that seem to come from the direction of the main beam, and refraction of the transmitted beam by interposed tissues can also give this effect.

Echocardiography equipment

Requirement for specialised equipment

Imaging the heart presents special challenges. The lungs and ribcage permit only limited access for reliable transmission of ultrasound energy. The cardiac chambers and valves are constantly in motion and thus temporal resolution is an important consideration. Analysis of blood flow patterns and pressure gradients is a critical diagnostic technique and high-quality Doppler imaging is important for accurate diagnosis. Improvements in ultrasound imaging techniques and computing technologies now mean that many 'ordinary' ultrasound machines can incorporate echocardiography simply by purchasing the appropriate analysis software, attaching a suitable transducer and activating the relevant operating profile.

Fundamental machine controls include a means of selecting the correct transducer and the desired imaging mode, controlling both the power of the transmitted ultrasound beam and the gain of the receiving amplifiers, and controlling the field depth. A keyboard and a means of permanently storing and archiving the study (live video and still frames) are also provided. A 'freeze' control will freeze the image on the screen and turn off the ultrasound transmission. Typically, several seconds of video will be retained in the memory and can be examined in freeze mode by using a scroll control. A cursor is used to measure distances or time intervals, and to trace areas. The ECG should be displayed on the screen to facilitate interpretation of observed events, and other physiological inputs may be offered, depending on the type of machine.

As well as the ultrasound image, the display will include patient details, technical information about the image, such as the transducer frequencies and screen refresh rate, and the current date and time. A speaker facility is often provided. Doppler frequencies (see later) are generally in the audible range, and the sound can help acquire an optimal trace.

Extensive processing takes place after the echoes have been detected by the transducer. Traditionally this has been divided into pre-processing (amplification and processing of the analogue signal) and post-processing (manipulation of the digital representation of the echo for the purposes of display).

After pre-processing, the amplitude of the echoes varies widely, with very faint echoes from red cells (which can be ignored if not in Doppler mode), loud echoes from highly reflective interfaces, and intermediate echoes from other tissues. It is this last group that is most of interest because a non-linear allocation of the echo amplitude to the grey-scale value stretches out these intermediate echoes, generally showing everything fainter as black, and everything louder as white.

As computing technology improves, the conversion from analogue to digital signal is generally moving closer to the transducer, and more of the processing is done by computer, blurring the distinction between pre- and post-processing. Experience and institutional wisdom

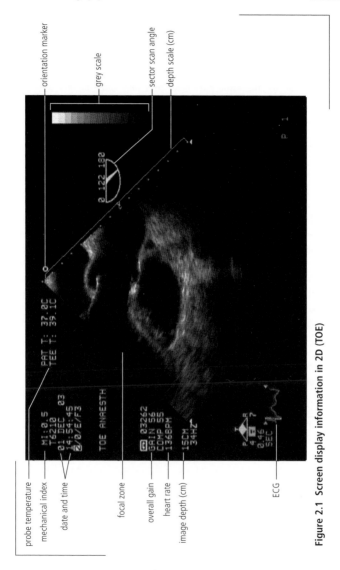

Figure 2.1 Screen display information in 2D (TOE)

will help select the best post-processing mode. Harmonic resonance imaging, which takes advantage of non-linearities in the transmission of sound through the tissues, giving rise to harmonics, is used to enhance contrast resolution. Different manufacturers may use different terms for the same parameter and may offer slightly different controls for manipulating image quality (see Chapter 3).

Imaging transducers

Transthoracic windows to the heart are available in the intercostal spaces at the apex and on either side in the parasternal region, from the subcostal/epigastric region and from the suprasternal notch. Transducers for TTE need to be small because of the limited size of these windows.

Imaging from the oesophagus or stomach (TOE) gives excellent views of many cardiac and major vascular structures, although the left main bronchus impedes imaging of the distal ascending aorta, proximal aortic arch and left pulmonary artery. The transducer of a TOE probe has to be small because it is mounted in a modified endoscope.

The solution to examining a large heart from a small window is to sweep a very narrow ultrasound beam from side to side, drawing the resulting pattern of echoes as bright spots on the corresponding points of the screen. This is why echocardiograph images typically have a 'sector' appearance; whether the origin of the sector is drawn at the top or the bottom of the screen is irrelevant. Older probes had a mechanical system for sweeping the sector, but most current systems use a 'phased array' to achieve directional control of the beam without requiring any moving parts.

The active part of the transducer consists of an array of piezoelectric elements. Each piezocrystal can act as an ultrasound source and detector, and can act independently of adjacent crystals. Phased-array transducers use staggered timing of the activation of each crystal to steer and focus the ultrasound beam in the required direction. Linear arrays are often used for transcutaneous or intraoperative vascular imaging, which produce a rectangular image on the screen. They have very high frequencies and excellent resolution, but are not well suited for general cardiac imaging. Considerable engineering ingenuity is employed to enhance the transfer of ultrasound energy between the transducer and the tissues. Specialised non-imaging CW Doppler probes are available, offering improved directionality and spectral purity.

Imaging modes

The standard imaging mode is 2D or B (brightness). A very short ping of ultrasound energy is emitted into the tissues and the transducer is then switched to 'listen' mode to detect the echoes. After sufficient time has passed to allow echoes from the current depth setting to return, the next ping is transmitted, slightly to the side of the first. Over subsequent pings the beam is scanned across the image sector; for example, for a 10-cm field depth, approximately 7500 pings are emitted every second.

M (motion) mode exchanges 2D image quality for high temporal resolution along a single line. All of the imaging pings are directed along the line of interest, rather than scanning through the imaging plane. Historically, M-mode predates the other imaging modes; the nomenclature of the movement of the mitral valve leaflets during the cardiac cycle is based on M-mode imaging. Phased-array transducers can commit alternate pings to M-mode and 2D mode, and permit simultaneous display of an M-mode image and a live 2D pilot view.

3D imaging uses ECG-gated acquisition of 2D images over a wide range of plane angles, either by rotating the transducer head or by using a 2D phased array. After the scan data is acquired, the 3D image is reconstructed and can be presented as a loop. Real-time (4D) imaging is now available on some machines.

Doppler effect and Doppler imaging modes

The Doppler effect is the change in the frequency of a wave when the observer is moving relative to the source. The Doppler frequency, f_D, is the frequency difference, and is proportional to the relative axial velocity of the source of the echo and the original emitted frequency f. In ultrasound imaging the effect is doubled because the moving subject produces an echo at its shifted frequency, and in turn the transducer observes the echo with the Doppler effect again applied:

$$f_D = 2fv\cos\theta$$

where v is the speed of the source of the echo and θ is the angle between the motion and the ultrasound beam. If flow occurs at right angles to the ultrasound beam, $\cos\theta = 0$ and there is no Doppler shift.

Red blood cells generate the echoes used for most Doppler studies. They are poor reflectors (showing black in 2D imaging modes), and high-power transmission and receiver amplifier gains are required, which results in a particular susceptibility to interference (such as from diathermy).

Three Doppler-based modes are used in echocardiography: pulse wave (PW), continuous wave (CW) and colour flow mapping (CFM, or Colour). Both PW and CW exchange 2D image quality for velocity information and the display shows the velocity spectrum on the vertical axis versus time on the horizontal axis. For both modes, a cursor sets the area to be processed: for CW this will be a line, and for PW it is be a spot (or spots) along the line.

The echocardiography machine uses a fast Fourier transform to extract frequency spectrum information from the echoes. High-amplitude, low-velocity signals are discarded and the resulting spectrum is displayed with the Doppler shift frequency automatically converted to velocity.

PW Doppler involves the transmission of pings along the line of interest. Analysis of the signal is gated so that only echoes arising from the cursor position are processed. A well-acquired PW trace of laminar flow shows a narrow band ('spectral purity'), whereas turbulent flow appears as a filled in, bidirectional envelope. The audio output from laminar flow is a clear whistling tone and turbulent flow has a harsh scratchy quality.

PW Doppler is subject to the Nyquist theorem, which limits the maximum detectable Doppler frequency depending on the pulse frequency. The Nyquist limit is the maximum velocity that can be unambiguously determined using PW Doppler. Velocities exceeding this limit are 'wrapped around' (i.e. aliasing) and appear as large velocities in the other direction. Experience will enable recognition of this phenomenon.

CW Doppler involves continuous transmission along the desired line, which is set by moving the relevant cursor. Some of the crystals in the transducer array are left in 'receive' mode' so that ultrasound transmission and reception occurs simultaneously. CW Doppler is used for measuring high velocities because it is not subject to the Nyquist limit, but ranging is not possible. A CW Doppler display can be recognised because the velocity envelope is always solidly filled in.

In CFM the Doppler shift information is superimposed on a 2D

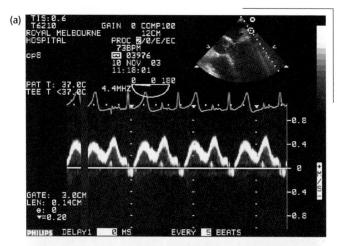

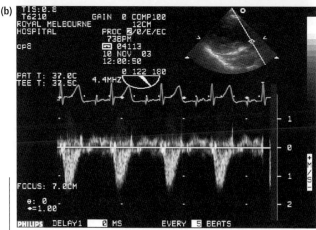

Figure 2.2 (a) Pulse wave Doppler in the left upper pulmonary vein (TOE). **(b)** Continuous wave Doppler through the aortic valve (TOE)

image. Several pings are required to analyse (by autocorrelation) each line in the colour sector, so temporal resolution is degraded, but this effect can be minimised by limiting the colour sector to the area of interest. CFM is also subject to Nyquist aliasing.

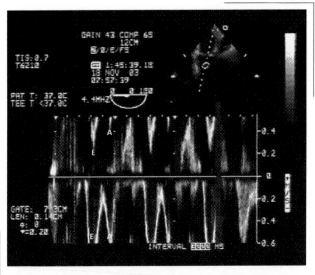

Figure 2.3 Mitral inflow Doppler exhibiting aliasing. Note that the peak E and A waves are wrapped around and displayed in the other channel because the Nyquist limit has been exceeded (TOE)

Colour M-mode combines CFM and M-mode and can be used in assessment of diastolic function. It is also possible to perform Doppler analysis of signals arising from the tissues (tissue Doppler imaging).

The role of Doppler imaging in echocardiography is discussed in more detail in Chapter 7.

Limitations in echocardiography

Electrical interference is a frequent problem in the operating theatre. Prosthetic valves or extensive valvular calcification can limit the available views. Reverberation and side-lobe artifact can appear remarkably compelling and it is not unknown for surgery to be performed on artifactual lesions.

Some limitations are fundamental to ultrasound imaging and arise from the physics and technology. The field depth is a particular consideration; it adversely impacts on temporal, spatial and contrast resolution because high-amplitude, relatively low-frequency pings are required. Field depth should be set to the lowest value that clearly shows the area of interest.

Poor reflections arise from interfaces parallel to the ultrasound beam, which can result in lateral wall dropout, making it difficult to define the endocardial borders of the septal and lateral walls of the left ventricle.

CFM degrades temporal resolution, and the colour sector should also be reduced to the minimum area consistent with adequate visualisation.

The Nyquist effect limits velocity (and therefore pressure) estimations in the pulsed Doppler modes (CFM and PW). Velocity determination of poorly aligned flows is subject to error even when an attempt is made to allow for the cosine of the relative angle.

Despite impressive developments in the applied technology of ultrasound, the final limitation will always be the operator. An unhurried, systematic approach and careful attention to optimisation of the image will minimise the risk of an important finding being missed.

Chapter 3
Obtaining the best image

Ruari Orme

Learning objectives
1. Understand the basic ultrasound machine controls.
2. Understand how to obtain the best image.
3. Understand the types of imaging artifacts.

Factors affecting the ultrasound image

Echocardiography is an 'operator dependent' investigation, which means that the information derived from a complete echocardiographic examination depends on the quality of the images the operator obtains and then analyses. Deductions made from poor quality images may result in an inappropriate course of management that could potentially lead to patient morbidity. Therefore, every effort should be made to optimise the image for evaluation.

There are three factors that have the greatest impact on image quality: the operator, the patient and the machine

Operator
The operator must understand three-dimensional anatomy, ultrasound physics, and pathology in order to generate clear, representative images and make real-time comments on the images obtained. The operator's skills must be kept up to date by regularly performing and reporting ultrasound examinations.

Patient

Both the patient's anatomy and the type of anaesthetic affect the quality of the ultrasound image. Anatomy may be rotated or distorted by cardiac or respiratory pathology, such as chronic obstructive airways disease, obesity or intrathoracic masses. Adequacy of sedation (for TOE) and positioning is important in the non-anaesthetised patient. Gas or food in the stomach will impair propagation of the sound beam. Care must be taken not to injure the patient while trying to get the perfect image; for example, avoid extreme anteflexion in the oesophagus during TOE.

Ultrasound machine

To obtain an adequate image the operator must consider the area of interest, depth, frame rate, ultrasound frequency, angle of insonation and the potential for artifacts. Using basic principles of ultrasound physics (see Chapter 2), knowledge of normal anatomy, and methodical persistence will assist in the acquisition of useful, replicable images. Familiarity with the dials and buttons on the machine ('knobology') also facilitates this process.

Instrument layout and settings

All ultrasound machines have a similar basic structure, but there are individual differences in appearance and terminology, so the operator should consult the manufacturer's handbook or company representative to ensure complete familiarity with a particular machine. The following is a basic introduction to the common dials, buttons and presets of a 'generic' ultrasound machine (Figures 3.1, 3.2). It is important to commence each ultrasound examination with appropriate labelling and machine set-up.

Commencement

Patient ID/ Begin	Enter the patient details to allow annotation of patient data on image for storage, retrieval and identification purposes.
Set-up	Enables the system to obtain physiological data, ECG, respiratory and pulse waveforms. Many machines have these preset.

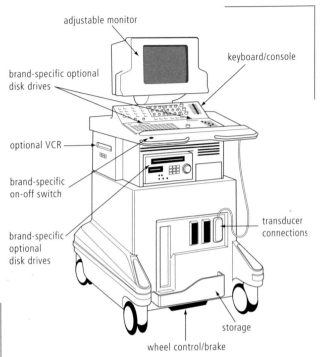

Figure 3.1 'Generic' ultrasound machine showing the controls on the keyboard as buttons and dials arranged in functional groups

Physio	Enables manipulation and display of physiological variables.
Study type	Enables selection of examination-specific control settings. The machine will have in-built initial settings for calculations package, gain, power, colour maps and compression to assist with general settings for the study (e.g. TOE vs TTE vs surface ultrasound vs vascular examinations).
Transducer	Enables choice of probe
Alphanumeric keyboard	Used to annotate the image with text, and for entry of patient details.

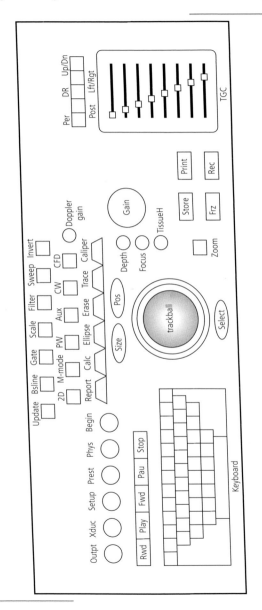

Figure 3.2 Keyboard controls

B mode/2D image tuning controls

Depth	Adjusts the vertical field of view: increasing the depth setting decreases the frame rate.
Size	Allows alteration of the size of the window of the region of interest using the trackball.
Position	Allows movement of the window of the ultrasound beam using the trackball.
Invert/ Up-Down	Changes the orientation of the image, displaying structures closest to the transducer at the bottom of the screen.
Left/Right	Changes the orientation of the image by reversing the image (mirror image).
Gain	Adjusts the acoustic power of the transmitted signals and the amplification of the received signals. Undergaining results in the loss of low-level echo signals; overgaining results in reduced contrast resolution and the increased possibility of artifacts in otherwise 'echo free' areas.
TGC	Sliders for adjusting the amplification of the returning signals according to depth are arranged in a vertical fashion.
Tissue H(armonics)	With the activation of tissue harmonics, the machine analyses returning echoes of higher harmonic frequencies, rather than the transmitted fundamental frequency. Sometimes this will 'clean up' a poor image by improving endocardial definition, but care must be taken in the 2D assessment of valves because they may appear thicker.
Compression/ Dynamic Range	Adjusts the dynamic range of returning echoes. Lowering the dynamic range removes from the display any weak echoes that may be attributable to acoustic noise; however, care must be taken to ensure information from interfaces reflecting low-level echoes is not lost.
Colour Grey Scale/B Colour	Unrelated to colour Doppler, it enables a choice of display of the 2D/B-mode image. The operator can select a shade of colour rather than using the standard grey scale, which may improve contrast resolution.

Focus/Focal Zone(s)	Usually depicted as a triangle or arrow on the display, the focal zone is the area at which the ultrasound beam is narrowest. It is within this area that the best lateral resolution can be obtained. It is therefore recommended to set the focal zone at the area of interest. Some systems have multiple focal zones available, which enhances lateral resolution at different depths, but the trade-off is a reduction in frame rate and the production of range ambiguity artifacts.
Zoom/Res	Activates a small adjustable 'box' that can be moved to the area of interest and then magnified without compromising spatial resolution.
Post processing/ Delta	Controls the degree of contrast resolution by reassigning different levels of grey to the amplitude of the returning echoes. The trade-off is the loss of contrast resolution between echoes from different interfaces that have been assigned the same shade.
Persist/Frame Averaging	Improves the signal-to-noise ratio by averaging the data from more than one frame. If required, decreasing the 'frame averaging' is recommended to reduce the loss of spatial resolution (image blurring) in a moving subject/tissue.

Mode controls

2D	Enables display and manipulation of real-time 2D images
M-mode	Enables display and manipulation of real-time one-dimensional images
PW	Activates pulse wave Doppler within the 2D image. The Doppler sample volume size and position can be adjusted with the trackball.
CW	Activates continuous wave Doppler within the 2D image. The Doppler beam/cursor is positioned with the trackball.
Blind CW/ Aux/Non 2D probe	Activates a separate 'blind' (non 2D) image. A CW probe is available on most systems and is used for more accurate assessment of Peak and

Mean velocities and gradients. Spectral Doppler waveform, timing in the cardiac cycle (ECG) and characteristic sounds are used as a guide to identify which valve or area of flow disturbance is being interrogated.

Colour   Activates a window of colour flow Doppler within the 2D image. Having a large CFD box over a large area of the 2D image decreases the frame rate and leads to jerky images, colour jets not being shown and artifactual blurring of objects. These artifacts can be minimised by reducing the width and depth of the colour sector using the size and position controls of the trackball. Generally, Blue is blood flowing Away from the transducer, Red is blood flowing Towards (BART).

Tissue   Once the cursor and sample volume are in place,
Doppler   activation of TDI (a form of PW) enables
Imaging   detection of the low-velocity, high-amplitude
(TDI)   echoes reflected from the mitral valve annulus or myocardium at a specific site. The velocities are more commonly displayed as PW Doppler waveforms.

Doppler and M-mode controls

Cursor   Usually a dotted or straight line, placed in the area of interest using the trackball when interrogating with M-mode or CW. When activated for PW or TDI it has a 'sample gate' (i.e. two horizontal lines or bracket tethered to the cursor).

Colourise   Unrelated to colour Doppler, it is the operator's preference for how the spectral Doppler or M-mode image is displayed. The operator can select a shade of colour rather than using the standard black/grey/white, which may improve visualisation.

Baseline   Horizontal line representing zero Doppler shift, which appears on the display when CW, PW or TDI are activated and is evident on the colour bar when CFD is activated. It may be lowered or raised depending on the direction of the blood flow of interest in order to display the complete spectral Doppler profile (unless significant aliasing is evident). Generally, blood flowing towards the transducer is displayed above the baseline, blood flowing away is displayed below the baseline. The CFD baseline may be altered in some circumstances, such as obtaining an aliased velocity for proximal isovelocity surface area (PISA) measurements.

Scale/Velocity In PW and CFD modes, this range is dependent upon the pulse repetition frequency. In PW, CW and TDI modes, it should be increased in order to display the complete spectral Doppler profile and decreased (provided it does not result in aliasing) to make the spectral Doppler profile larger for measuring purposes. The CFD scale may be adjusted to improve visualisation of the blood flow: decrease the CFD scale in areas of low flow and decrease the depth/colour box size in order to increase the scale in areas of high-velocity flow. Altering the scale (distance) in M-mode involves adjusting the overall depth.

Filter Removes from the spectral Doppler display any low-velocity, high-amplitude echoes that are assumed to be generated by vessel walls and moving cardiac tissue. Care must be taken in setting the filter so that clean Doppler profiles are displayed without eliminating significant low-flow velocities.

Sweep Decreasing the sweep speed enables visualisation of more cardiac cycles on the display during PW, CW, TDI or M-modes, which may be useful when assessment of the variations between cycles is necessary (e.g. ventricular interdependence when using M-mode or respiratory variation when using PW). Increasing the sweep speed enables for more accurate measurements to be done.

Update Present on some systems, a small, real-time image is displayed while in a particular mode, which enables the operator to reposition the cursor.

Invert	Changes the orientation of the Doppler profile on the display. The actual direction of blood flow should be noted.
Colour Doppler Gain	Changes the amplification of the colour Doppler echo signals. It is recommended to initially 'overgain' the area of interest by increasing the Colour gain to the level at which the colour has a 'speckled' appearance, then decrease it slightly to the level at which this does not occur.
M-mode Gain	The overall 2D/B-mode gain control that can be adjusted while in M-mode.
Spectral Doppler Gain	Changes the amplification of the spectral Doppler signals. It should be set at the level at which the waveform appears 'clean' (i.e. without noise). 'Overgaining' affects the height of the waveform and can result in erroneous peak velocity measurements.
Gate/Sample Size/Sample Volume	Length of time and therefore the depth from which Doppler signals are received and analysed in PW mode. It may need to be adjusted when alternating between sites of interrogation and modes (e.g. PW vs TDI). It is recommended that the sample volume be kept as small as possible to reduce the occurrence of spectral broadening. Note that when High PRF is activated (increasing the PW scale/PRF to increase the Nyquist limit), two or more sample gates may be present, in which case it is recommended that the extra sample gate(s) are in 'no/low flow' areas to decrease range ambiguity.

Measurements and trackball controls

Trackball	Enables control of the size and positioning of the Doppler, M-mode and text cursors and the 2D and colour flow Doppler windows, as well as scrolling through frozen images.
Freeze	Creates a static image for further analysis. Leftward or rightward rotation of the trackball will allow scrolling through images.

Analysis/ Calculations	Enables calculation of derived indices such as dimensions, area volumes, and masses, depending on the installed software.
Enter	Upon completion of analysis of a frozen image, pressing the enter key will allow manipulation and further analysis of the same frame or other frames.
Trace	Activates a cursor on the image. Press it again and rotation of the trackball enables the operator to circumscribe the area of the region of interest.
Caliper	Activates a cursor on the image. Press it again and rotation of the trackball enables a distance to be generated between two areas of interest.
Erase	Removal of erroneous traces or calipers.

Archive controls

Disk	Storage and retrieval from optical disk.
VCR controls	Storage and retrieval from videotape (e.g. Tape/ Record: press this key to commence VCR recording).
Acquire/ Store/Loop	Stores colour, real-time or frozen images.
Print	Hardcopy generation of acquired image via built-in printer.
Report	Displays data from the measurements performed during the current study.

Room configuration

The operator of the ultrasound machine should also consider the environment in which the examination is taking place. Lighting, patient positioning, surgical and ergonomic factors will all affect image quality. Ideally, the patient should be in a comfortable, supported position, with ambient lighting reduced to enhance the image. Diathermy impairs image quality. In a busy operating theatre obtaining ideal conditions may be difficult!

The operator should be in a position to manipulate the transducer and have one hand free to use the machine controls. Figure 3.3 is a diagram of the arrangement of our operating theatre. Note the

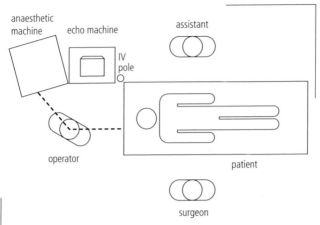

Figure 3.3 Suggested room configuration. Note the operator is using the right hand for probe manipulation and the left for control adjustment. Note also that an IV pole is used to suspend the TOE probe handle for ease of use.

position of the operator at the head of the patient facing the ultrasound monitor, with the anaesthetic machine in view to the left. It is important (if the operator is the anaesthetist) that the anaesthetic monitors, the patient and the echocardiography machine are all in the same visual sector.

Artifacts and pitfalls

Poor image quality and difficulty in obtaining a representative image are not the only causes of an inadequate ultrasound examination. Misinterpretation of an adequate image may also occur if the operator is unfamiliar with potential imaging artifacts and pitfalls.

Artifacts

An artifact occurs when the image generated by the ultrasound beam does not represent the actual physical structure being examined. Artifacts include the appearance of a structure that does not exist or failure to present an image of a structure that is present. Artifacts are not bound by tissue planes and will often cross anatomical borders. They may also disappear or change sites when viewed from another angle. Artifacts will not appear closer to the probe than the structure that produces them, thus they will appear at the same depth or more.

Artifacts encountered during routine scanning are attributable to the conflict between the assumptions made by the machine of the nature of the ultrasound being emitted and received, and the inherent variables of the subject being scanned.

Ultrasound system assumptions

- The speed of sound in soft tissue is 1540 m/s.
- All echoes received have originated from the beam centre.
- Ultrasound beams propagate and return in a straight line.
- The loss of echo intensity is constant throughout the imaging sector.
- The depth of a structure is calculated from the time it takes for a transmitted echo to return to the transducer.

Pitfalls

A pitfall is a normal cardiac structure (or variant) that is presumed by an inexperienced operator to be pathology (e.g. thrombus, tumour or endocarditis). Experience, knowledge of anatomy and understanding of the ultrasound representation of that anatomy will reduce the risk of failing to recognise normal structures.

Common pitfalls

Atrial variants

'Coumarin' ridge	Ridge between the left atrial appendage and left upper pulmonary vein. It can be large, extending to the fossa ovalis, and often mistaken for thrombus, resulting in inappropriate warfarin therapy (Figure 3.4).
Atrial appendage lobes	Variation in the number of lobes in the left atrium is common and bands caused as a result of multilobed atrial appendages may be mistaken for thrombus (Figure 3.5).

Eustachian valve	Embryological remnant forming a ridge (or flap) of tissue that extends specifically from the border of the inferior vena cava and right atrium (Figure 3.6).
Chiari network	Filamentous embryological remnant in the right atrium, usually originating from a Eustachian valve, found in 8% of the population. It may be classified as pathological if it obstructs flow from the inferior vena cava or flow through the tricuspid valve (Figure 3.7).
Crista terminalis	Muscular ridge originating from the border of the superior vena cava and right atrium is linear in shape, but may still be mistaken for thrombus (Figure 3.8).

Ventricular variants

| Moderator band | Only seen in the right ventricle, this muscular band originates from the ventricular septum (septal band of the crista supraventricularis). It is useful for recognising the right ventricle in certain congenital heart diseases (Figure 3.9). |
| Left ventricular false tendons | 2–3 mm bands crossing the left ventricle and not contracting or thickening during systole. False tendons are generally benign, but may form abnormal conducting tracts allowing re-entrant ventricular tachycardias (Figure 3.10). |

Valvular variants

| Lambl's excrescences | Age-related fibrous strands that commonly originate from a nodule of Arantius, and are not more than 1 mm thick and 10 mm long. Differentiated from endocarditis by not having independent motion, being small and no associated valvular regurgitation. Excrescences longer than 10 mm should be considered pathological (fibroelastoma) (Figure 3.11). |

Septal variants

| Lipomatous hypertrophy | Fatty thickening of the atrial septum, not involving the fossa ovalis, that has an 'hourglass' or 'dumb-bell' appearance. It may be confused with other infiltrative processes such as amyloid (Figure 3.12). |
| Atrial septal aneurysm | Septal motion greater than 1.5 cm during the cardiac cycle, associated with an increased risk of stroke (Figure 3.13). |

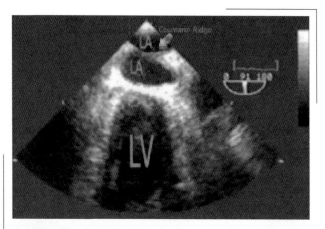

Figure 3.4 Coumarin ridge

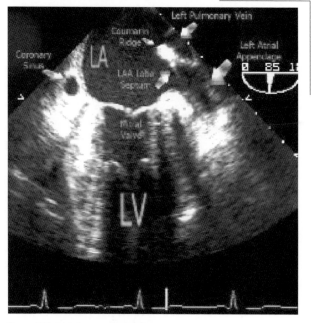

Figure 3.5 Atrial appendage lobe

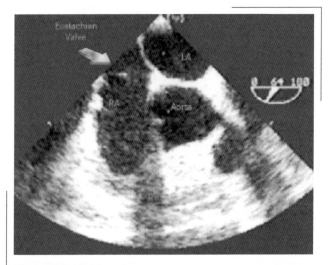

Figure 3.6 Eustachian valve

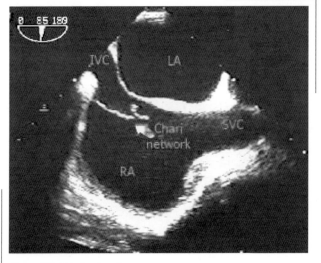

Figure 3.7 Chiari network

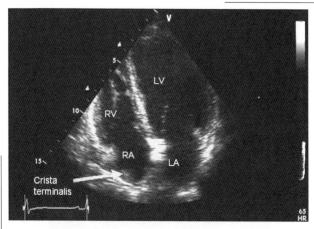

Figure 3.8 Crista terminalis

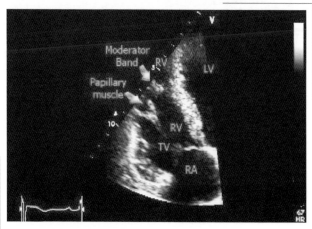

Figure 3.9 Moderator band

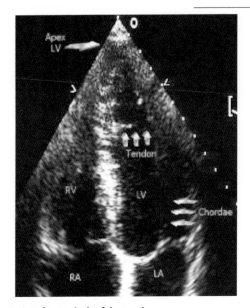

Figure 3.10 Left ventricular false tendons

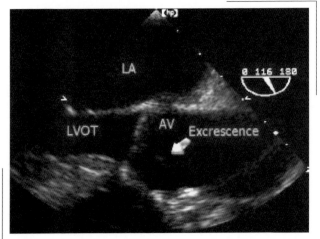

Figure 3.11 Lambl's excresences

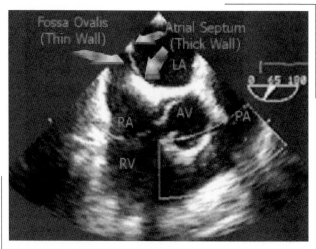

Figure 3.12 Lipomatous hypertrophy

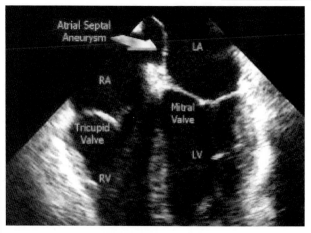

Figure 3.13 Atrial septal aneurysm

Chapter 4

Core anatomy for echocardiography

Alistair Royse

Learning objectives
1. Understand general cardiac anatomy.
2. Learn cardiac anatomy by memorising 2D echocardiography 'slices'.
3. Understand the regional relational anatomy of the heart, oesophagus and chest wall.
4. Understand variations in anatomy that may affect image quality.

Overview of thoracic anatomy

Echocardiographers need to understand basic cardiac anatomy and the relational anatomy of the heart, oesophagus, pleura and chest wall.

The heart lies behind the body of the sternum, and the aortic arch and its branches lie behind the manubrium. The diaphragm lies in a horizontal plane at the level of the sixth costal cartilage and 10 cm superior to the inferior extent of the xiphisternum.

Transthoracic echocardiography uses a window that is lateral to the sternum but medial to the pleural reflection of the contained lung (Figure 4.1). Costal cartilage will degrade the quality of the image, particularly if there is calcification, so the pleural reflection is most important.

The pleural reflection is attached to the sternum and the pericardium. Between these two attachments, the pleura can expand if the lungs are hyperinflated from chronic airways disease. On the right side, the sternal pleura attaches near the midline (Figure 4.1). The pericardial attachment reflects the sternal attachment and so the lung normally lies anterior to the right atrium. On the left, the sternal pleural attachment lies near the midline in the upper chest and at the fourth costal cartilage it then diverts laterally in an oblique line to the sixth costal cartilage. The pericardial attachment of the pleura also diverts at the same level and lies halfway between the midline and the lateral extent of the pericardium.

When the lungs are hyperinflated because of chronic airways disease, it is common to observe both lungs meeting or even crossing the midline. Consequently, the space between the pericardium and the chest wall will be entirely occupied by lung, which results in very poor TTE images.

The oesophagus lies in the posterior mediastinum with the trachea and right and left main bronchi lying between it and the great vessels. The gastro-oesophageal junction is usually 40 cm from the teeth. In the superior third of the thorax, the oesophagus lies slightly to the left; in the central portion, the aortic arch is present and the oesophagus is moved towards the right. If a hiatus hernia is present, it will most commonly be the sliding type and appears to have little effect on image quality. Less is known of the effect of other oesophageal or para-oesophageal types of hernia on image quality.

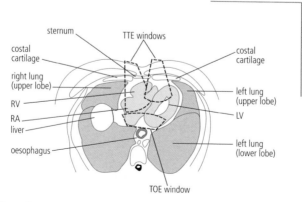

Figure 4.1 Acoustic windows for TTE and TOE

Perforations of the oesophagus by the probe will occur in the lower oesophagus, almost invariably where it turns anteriorly and to the left as it passes over the descending aorta, with the probe perforating the right side while taking a straight course. Typically, the patient is elderly with comorbidities such as renal failure, malnutrition or steroid use, which contribute to the tissue having poor tensile strength.

In the upper half of the chest, the trachea and then the right main bronchus is present anterior to the oesophagus, obstructing views of the proximal aortic arch and right brachiocephalic and common carotid arteries (Figure 4.2) because the air in the structures prevents transmission of the ultrasound. On the left lies the subclavian artery, and the distal aortic arch can be seen. In the lower half of the chest, the structures anterior to the oesophagus include the ascending aorta, right pulmonary artery, superior vena cava, left atrium and inferior vena cava (Figure 4.3). The size of the acoustic window is limited by the left and right main bronchi. Other structures of the heart lie obliquely and to the left of the oesophagus. Immediately to the left of the oesophagus, lies the descending aorta.

The inferior wall of the heart lies against the diaphragm, which in turn lies against the fundus of the stomach and sometimes the left lobe of the liver. The visible structures include the inferior extent of the right ventricle and the inferior wall of the left ventricle. The long-axis

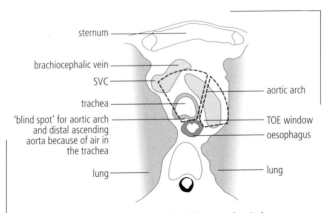

Figure 4.2 Effect of the trachea on the TOE acoustic window

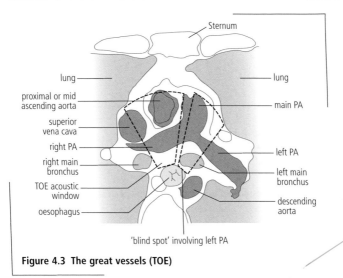

Figure 4.3 The great vessels (TOE)

of the left ventricle, however, is often directed inferior to the horizontal plane on the left side. Consequently, the plane of the long-axis of the left ventricle and that adopted by the echocardiography probe will frequently not be parallel.

Overview of cardiac anatomy

Base of the heart and valves

The term 'base' of the heart is confusing. Anatomy students frequently refer to the four pulmonary veins entering the left atrium, where the pericardium is reflected around the anterior and lateral aspects of the veins and the atrium, including the posterior aspect of the left atrium between the veins (oblique sinus). The heart is restrained posteriorly by these attachments.

Surgeons, however, frequently refer to the base of the heart as the fibrous skeleton of the heart (Figure 4.4), which lies in an oblique plane approximating the left axilla and the right iliac crest. In this plane, the four valves are present and, externally, the atrioventricular groove. The aortic valve lies centrally, with the pulmonary valve anterior and to the left. Posterior and to the left lies the mitral valve, and

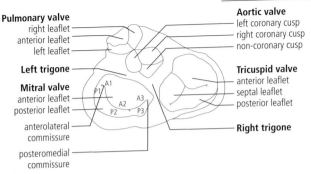

Figure 4.4 Relationship between the cardiac valves and the fibrous skeleton

to the right the tricuspid valve. The annuli of the mitral and tricuspid valves merge to form the fibrous skeleton of the heart with a membranous septum. The central portion is a fibrous body that has two extensions.

The fibrous skeleton is, however, not a flat plane and so each of the four valves lie in a slightly different plane and have a different angulation to the other valves. Therefore, it is not possible to view all the valves from one position or with a single angle of rotation of the probe.

The mitral valve has a larger anterior leaflet and the posterior leaflet occupies the posterior two-thirds of the annulus and is subject to annular dilatation. The conventional echocardiographic description of this valve follows that of Carpentier. The letter 'A' refers to the anterior leaflet and 'P' to the posterior leaflet. Adjacent to this letter is a number corresponding to the three segments of the posterior leaflet as described by Ranganathan et al. Alternatively these segments are referred to as scallops. '1' refers to that part of the valve closest to the left atrial appendage, or the left or lateral side of the valve when seen directly through the left atrium; '3' refers to the side of the valve closest to the right atrium and coronary sinus or medial side; '2' refers to the central portion of the leaflet. The orifice of the left atrial appendage lies near P1 (lateral scallop), that of the circumflex artery near P1 and P2 (middle scallop) and for the coronary sinus near P3 (medial scallop).

The tricuspid valve has a large anterior leaflet, a relatively small septal leaflet that lies posteriorly and along the tendon of Todaro, and a small posterior leaflet that lies inferiorly. The aortic and pulmonary valves are structurally very similar; both have three leaflets and the base of each leaflet is elliptical in shape. The Sinuses of Valsalva are dilated pockets of the aortic or pulmonary root adjacent to each of the leaflets. The aortic valve has a right coronary cusp that lies anteriorly and opposite the right coronary artery. The left coronary cusp lies posteriorly and to the left and opposite the left coronary artery. The non-coronary cusp lies posteriorly and to the right, and is adjacent to the roof of the left and right atria.

Coronary arteries

The left main coronary artery arises from the middle of the Sinus of Valsalva of the left coronary cusp, posterior to the main pulmonary artery. The anterolateral branch is the left anterior descending artery, and branches from this vessel are referred to as diagonal arteries. The posterior branch is the circumflex artery and its branches are referred to as marginal arteries. Sometimes there is a relatively large branch of the left coronary artery between the circumflex and left anterior descending arteries, and it is referred to as the intermediate artery. The right coronary artery arises from the middle of the Sinus of Valsalva of the right coronary cusp, and travels anteriorly for a short distance before travelling inferiorly along the atrioventricular groove adjacent to the right atrium. It supplies the free right ventricular wall with branches called the acute marginal arteries, then divides into the posterior descending artery, which meets the left anterior descending artery at the apex of the left ventricle, and the left ventricular branch artery, which supplies the posterolateral aspect of the left ventricle.

The usual coronary anatomy comprises a large right coronary artery that has both posterior descending and left ventricular branch arteries, and this is referred to as a right dominant system (Figure 4.5). In less than 10% of patients, these two terminal branches will arise from a very large circumflex artery, with the right coronary artery supplying only the free right ventricular wall, and this is referred to as a left dominant system.

The ventricular septum is supplied by branches from both the left anterior descending artery and the posterior descending artery, and these are referred to as the septal branches.

Figure 4.6 shows the distribution of the coronary arteries.

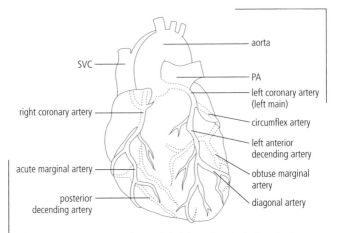

Figure 4.5 Coronary arteries and their branches (anterior view)

Ventricles

The left ventricle is elliptical in shape with the mitral valve at its base. Two papillary muscles, the anterolateral and posteromedial, are present in the mid segment. In dilated cardiomyopathy, the ventricle may have a more globular or spherical shape.

The right ventricle has a complex, triangular shape that is normally approximately two-thirds of the size of the left ventricle on the echocardiography image. In 60% of patients there is a prominent muscular band known as the moderator band. The annulus of the tricuspid valve is in plane with that of the mitral valve.

Segments of the left ventricle: The left ventricle is divided into three short-axis slices (basal, mid and distal/apical) that incorporate 16 segments plus the 17th segment or apical cap (Figure 4.6). A wall motion score is entered for each segment and a total score derived (see table in Figure 4.6).

Cardiac anatomy in echocardiography 'slices'

It will be some time before 3D images are widely available, so the simplest way to learn the regional anatomy seen on 2D echocardiography is to memorise the series of standard 'slices' or views that have been determined as representative of a good study and consider these

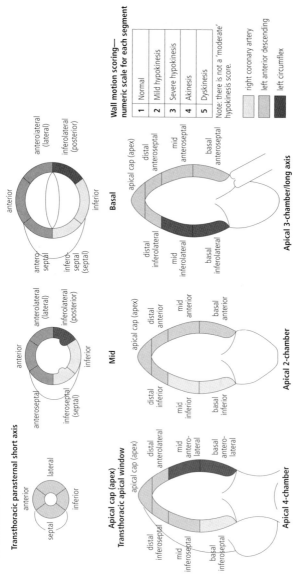

Figure 4.6 Seventeen-segment model of the left ventricle showing the coronary artery distribution

as 'snapshots' of the heart. Greater experience will enable recognition of variations from these standard views. It is important to realise that these views have been empirically determined by previous echocardiographers and reflect the constraints imposed by the 'window' of the probe, the echocardiographic lucency of the tissue being penetrated in the area of interest, and the echocardiography technology available at the time, including the probe configurations and frequency as well as the software and speed of computing hardware in the machine.

Variations in individual anatomy and implications for echocardiography

Have you often wondered why there is a range of probe positions and angles of rotation needed to achieve the same image in different patients? The answer is that the heart is not in the same position in all patients.

It is not entirely clear why such individual anatomical variation should occur. Nevertheless it highlights a most important point. Regional left ventricular walls are named according to the relative anatomy and not by the absolute relational anatomy. In other words, the anterior wall of the left ventricle is described as anterior because of its relationship to the interventricular septum. Therefore, the anterior wall retains its name even if it lies in a true lateral position in the patient's chest because of axial rotation of the heart.

Rotation in the sagittal plane
The heart is restrained posteriorly by the four pulmonary veins and anteriorly by the great vessels. Hence the heart may rotate around this base in the sagittal plane, most commonly to the 'left', which refers to a superior and left lateral displacement of the apex of the heart, causing the axis of the left ventricle to become more horizontal, rather than the inferior and oblique orientation normally seen. Any elongation of the ascending aorta then displaces the central and right side of the heart inferiorly onto the diaphragm, forcing a superior displacement of the left ventricular apex. An 'unfolded' aorta seen in the elderly and aortic aneurysms are examples of elongation of the aorta.

There may be elevation of the apex of the left ventricle when there is relative elevation of the diaphragm, caused by obesity, a thick-set or 'stocky' body shape, raised intraabdominal pressure from gastric or intestinal distension, ascites, or pregnancy. Loss of lung volume with pulmonary collapse, previous lung resection or phrenic nerve injury may also cause this variation. The heart may also be rotated in the opposite direction, to the 'right'; that is, the axis of the left ventricle is more vertical in the chest, which will usually occur with depression of the left hemidiaphragm related to chronic airways disease.

The implications of rotation to the left are diminished views of the left ventricle, particularly the apex, because it has been separated from the diaphragm, presumably by a lung interposed between the diaphragm and the pericardium. Rotation to the right, however, should improve transoesophageal imaging of this part of the heart. Rotation may also affect visualisation of the valves, with variable degrees of rotation of the probe required to obtain a standard image or view. In particular, the deep gastric view of the aortic valve may be affected with rotation of the heart to the left.

Rotation about the long axis of the heart

Normally, the left anterior descending artery adopts a course that is anterolateral and inferior to the horizontal. The most common form of rotation appears to be an anticlockwise rotation when seen from the right-hand side of the patient; that is, the left anterior descending artery lies in a more left and lateral position than normal. Consequently, the right ventricle has an entirely anterior and sometimes anterolateral position within the chest. In extreme cases, the left anterior descending artery may indeed lie in a true lateral position. Less commonly, the rotation along the long axis appears in the opposite direction, causing the left anterior descending artery to lie in a true anterior position.

Echocardiography 'blind spots'

Left ventricular apex (Figure 4.1)

The left ventricular apex may be very difficult to image when the heart is rotated to the left because there will be separation of the tissues between the heart, the diaphragm and the fundus of the stomach. Transthoracic 4-chamber views may also be difficult because of imposition of part of the lingula lobe of the left lung between the chest wall and pericardium.

Proximal aortic arch and distal ascending aorta (Figure 4.2)

The distal trachea and proximal right main bronchus lie between the oesophagus and the aortic structures, and the air within them prevents transmission of the ultrasound signal, which is important during cardiac surgery because these sites are frequently manipulated for aortic cannulation during cardiac pulmonary bypass and aortic clamping. Atheroma in this area may be dislodged, causing atheroembolism.

Pulmonary artery bifurcation and left pulmonary artery, proximal superior vena cava (Figure 4.3)

The left main bronchus lies between the oesophagus and the left main pulmonary artery and the distal pulmonary artery trunk.

Left ventricle following prosthetic valve replacement or severe calcified mitral valve annulus

Oesophageal views of the left ventricle would normally pass through the mitral valve annulus, and views of the left ventricular outflow tract may also normally pass through the aortic valve annulus. Consequently, a prosthetic valve in the aortic or mitral position, or severe calcification, will prevent adequate imaging of the structures.

Chapter 5

Standard transoesophageal echocardiography examination

Joan Sutherland and Garry Donnan

Learning objectives
1. Understand the correct care of the TOE probe.
2. Understand how to conduct the standard TOE examination.

Care of the probe

Damaging the probe used for TOE can be expensive, but is easily avoided by ensuring that all operators undergo rigorous training programs, competency testing and ongoing monitoring. Practices outside the specifications recommended by the manufacturer will not be covered by warranty, in particular cuts, bites and abrasions to the probe.

Storage
The carry case is only for transportation of the probe, which should be stored in a secure location and not exposed to direct sunlight or extremes of temperature. The distal tip should be straight and

protected. The steering mechanism may be damaged if the flexible shaft is coiled into a diameter of less than 30 cm. Bite guards are recommended for use in all patients. The probe may also be damaged by autoclaving or leaving it in the cleaning or disinfection solution for longer than recommended. Prior to each use the probe must be examined carefully for damage and correct operation of the steering mechanism.

There are no exposed conductive surfaces distal to the control housing of the probe. If the outer layer of the shaft is damaged, the patient's oesophagus could be exposed to chassis leakage current and burnt. A combination of failure in the outer layer of the transducer sheath and in the electrosurgical unit may allow electrosurgical currents to return along the transducer conductor, also resulting in burns to the patient. Cardiac pacemakers are rarely a problem, but if interference does occur the echocardiography machine should be turned off immediately.

Cleaning and disinfection

Cleaning removes all the organic matter and other residues from the probe shaft, and should be carried out immediately after use so that secretions do not dry on the probe. The probe should be rinsed under running water, wiped with a soft cloth and soaked in enzymatic cleaner to remove all proteinaceous material. High-level disinfection using either glutaraldehyde-based or non-glutaraldehyde disinfectants kills bacteria, viruses and fungi. Bleach, acetone, Freon, hydrogen peroxide, ethylene oxide or heat sterilisation should not be used. Detailed records should be kept of probe cleaning and inspection.

The standard examination

The relative risks and benefits of TOE (i.e. probe insertion) must always be considered. If there is doubt a surgeon or a gastroenterologist should be consulted.

Absolute contraindications to TOE probe insertion and examination include:
- Presence of a vascular ring or active upper gastrointestinal bleeding
- Tracheo-oesophageal fistula or known perforated hollow viscus

- Oesophageal stricture or obstruction
- Unstable cervical spine
- Patient refusal.

Relative contraindications to probe insertion include:

- Oesophageal varices
- Barrett's oesophagus
- Zenker's diverticulum
- Oesophageal deformity
- Previous gastric or oesophageal surgery
- History of mediastinal radiation
- Severe coagulopathy
- Symptomatic hiatus hernia.

The TOE probe should be well lubricated and gently inserted into the oesophagus in the midline. Excessive force must never be used and all attempts abandoned if the probe does not pass easily. The probe should always be straight when it is moved in and out of the oesophagus. The safety of probe insertion is comparable to that of upper gastrointestinal endoscopy and has a reported morbidity of serious complications between 1:1000 and 1:5000 insertions. Lip trauma, dental damage and oesophageal injury, including perforation and vocal cord injuries, have been reported.

Basic manoeuvres

The operator must understand the basic manoeuvres of the probe, which are summarised in Figure 5.1. The large wheel controls ante-flexion and retroflexion. The small wheel controls flexion to the right and left. The TOE image is usually displayed with the near field at the top of the display.

Sector rotation is controlled by a button on the console. At 0° of rotation the right-hand side of the patient is seen on the left-hand side of the display, and the left side of the patient to the right of the display. Axial rotation of a multiplane probe from the horizontal plane (at 0°) towards the vertical plane (at 90°) is called 'forward rotation', and rotation in the opposite direction (90° to 0°) is 'backward rotation' or 'rotating back'.

Once a structure has been centred on the screen in one image plane, it will remain in the centre during rotations through to 180°, which enables the operator to obtain many views of a chosen structure, assisting in more accurate diagnosis. The abbreviations 'SAX' and 'LAX' refer to 'short axis' and 'long axis' respectively; for

From patient's view *Rotation forward*
is clockwise and moves from 0° to 180°
Rotation backward moves in the opposite direction

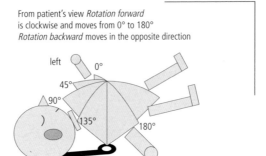

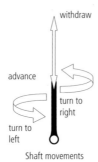

Shaft movements
using operator's hand

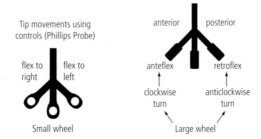

Tip movements using
controls (Phillips Probe)

Small wheel   Large wheel

Figure 5.1 Sector rotation and probe manoeuvres

example, the SAX view of the aortic valve shows the leaflets en face and the LAX shows a cross-section through the valve. The LAX view of the left ventricle refers to particular views in which both the mitral and the aortic valves are seen.

Basic views

The basic TOE examination recommended by the Society of Cardio-vascular Anesthesiologists and the American Society of Echocardio-graphy comprises 20 standard views. As shown in Figure 5.2 the TOE 'street map' uses names to assist recognition of the pathways to each of the standard views, but as the relationship of the oesophagus to the heart varies from patient to patient the same view may be found at slightly different locations. The map also shows the distances from the mouth to the different views, and diagrams of the probe's location and approximate beam direction.

Before starting the examination the machine controls must be adjusted and the sector depth chosen. In some clinical situations it may be prudent to proceed directly to the particular region of inter-est; however, whenever possible a comprehensive stepwise examina-tion should be performed because it will assist in the development of a thorough technique. Operator routine, of course, may vary and all approaches are acceptable, but each should aim to gather maximum information with minimum probe manipulation. Each structure is seen in more than one view. Probe position is described as upper-oesophageal (UO: 20–30 cm from the mouth), mid-oesophageal (MO: 30–40 cm) or transgastric (TG: below the diaphragm at a dis-tance of 40–50 cm). The deep TG view is found at 50 cm.

The standard views are numbered on the map from 1 to 20. At the top of the map is a rotation guide to each view (the 'street number'). Non-standard views are represented by letters and are all found on 'Main Street'.

Main Street is the pathway straight down the oesophagus to the stomach with no turns or rotations. There are five points of probe rota-tion to side streets, which are named according to the structures seen:

- Aortic Valve Avenue
- 4-Chamber Road and 4-Chamber Road West
- Ascending Aorta Road
- Dancing Donut Drive
- SA Mitral Street

  The sequence of the examination is as follows.

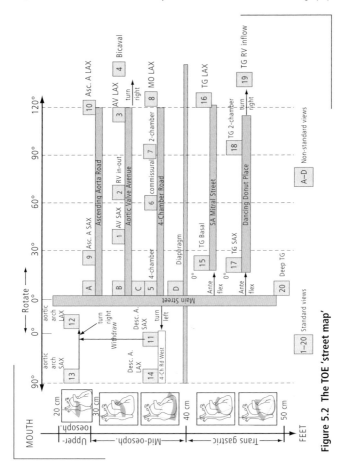

Figure 5.2 The TOE 'street map'

1. Aortic Valve Avenue

It is convenient to begin with the MO views at the level of the aortic valve (Figure 5.3: Aortic Valve Avenue). The short-axis view (MO AV SAX) is easy to find (view 1) by rotating to 30–40°. It is important that all three commissures of the aortic valve are identified. Next, rotate to 60–80° to obtain the right ventricular inflow–outflow view (MO RV inflow-outflow) (view 2), then the long-axis view (MO AV LAX) is obtained by rotating to 120°, ensuring that the left ventricular outflow tract (LVOT), aortic valve and aortic root are all seen (view 3). Next, turn the probe to the right to visit the bicaval view (MO bicaval) (view 4). To see the superior vena cava (SVC) more clearly, withdraw the probe; to identify the inferior vena cava (IVC) it may be necessary to advance the probe.

2. 4-Chamber Road

Once Aortic Valve Avenue is completed, proceed to 4-Chamber Road (Figure 5.4) by advancing the probe (with the probe tip straightened). The four cardiac chambers can be seen (MO 4 chamber) (view 5) with 10–15° of rotation required to optimise the view. From this probe position, move to 60° rotation to see the mitral commissures (MO mitral commissural). The chordal attachments of both papillary muscles are seen (view 6). Further rotation to 90° finds the mid-oesophageal 2-chamber view (MO 2 chamber) with the anterior left ventricular wall to the right of the screen, and the inferior wall to the left (view 7). At 120° is the mid-oesophageal long-axis view (MO LAX). There is a long-axis view of the aorta (view 8) and the adjacent anterior mitral valve leaflet. This completes 4-Chamber Road. The two non-standard views are the 5-chamber (withdraw slightly on the probe at 0°) and coronary sinus views (advance the probe at 0° until the coronary sinus comes into view).

3. Ascending Aorta Road

Although the ascending aortic views could be identified first (Figure 5.3), it is probably easier to do so after visiting 4-Chamber Road. The mid-oesophageal short-axis view (MO asc. aortic SAX) is located by withdrawing the probe a few centimetres and adding slight anteflexion of the probe if required (view 9). From this position adding a further 90° (to 120° rotation) locates the mid-oesophageal long-axis view (MO asc. aortic LAX) (view 10).

4. 4-Chamber Road West

To assess the aorta (Figure 5.5), with the probe at 0° and straight, withdraw to the MO 4-chamber view. Now turn the probe to the left and the circular descending aorta will be seen. The short-axis (MO desc. aorta SAX) (view 11) can also be rotated to 90° to examine the descending aorta in the long-axis (MO desc. aorta LAX) (view 14). Withdrawing the probe slowly from view 11 while turning it to the left reveals the long-axis view of the upper-oesophageal aortic arch (UO aortic arch LAX) (view 12). Finally, rotation to 90° displays the main pulmonary artery and pulmonary valve, with the aorta and the origin of the left subclavian artery at the top of the screen (UO aortic arch SAX) (view 13).

5. Transgastric views

Rotate back to 0° and advance the probe down Main Street into the stomach. Anteflexion of the probe locates the mid short-axis view (TG mid SAX) (view 17) at 0°, which has been termed the 'dancing donut', hence 'Dancing Donut Drive' (Figure 5.6). Here the two papillary muscles (anterolateral and posteromedial) are seen in cross-section. The inferior left ventricle is near the transducer (top of screen) and the anterior wall is at the bottom of the screen. The lateral wall is right of the screen and the interventricular septum is to the left.

From the TG mid SAX, rotate to 90° and visit the 2-chamber view (TG 2 chamber) (view 18) that shows the inferior left ventricular wall at the top of the screen and the anterior wall below. Turn the probe to the right and rotate to 120° and find the right ventricular inflow (TG RV inflow) (view 19). Further anteflexion of the probe from TG mid SAX reaches the basal short-axis view (TG basal SAX) (view 15), which is useful for assessing mitral valve function (SA Mitral Street). Rotation to 120° reveals the long-axis view (TG LAX) (view 16), which shows the LVOT and aortic valve. Advancing the probe further into the stomach at 0° (beyond Dancing Donut Drive) and further anteflexing the probe tip locates the deep long-axis view (deep TG LAX) (view 20) with the aortic valve in the far field (bottom of screen).

When a basic examination sequence has been developed, it can then be varied to meet particular clinical circumstances. Familiarity with the 20 basic views is essential, and additional brief comments about each of them are provided here.

1. MO AV SAX—The non-coronary cusp is opposite the interatrial septum. The origins of the coronary arteries can be seen when the probe is withdrawn slightly. Aortic valve area can be measured by planimetry.

2. MO RV inflow–outflow—Can assess both tricuspid valve and pulmonary valve disease, and get an indication of right ventricular function. Observe the passage of a pulmonary artery catheter.

3. MO AV LAX—Measure proximal aorta dimensions and assess aortic valve regurgitation using CFD.

4. MO bicaval—Useful for examining the interatrial septum for patent foramen ovale; the SVC, IVC and right atrial appendage can be seen.

5. MO 4-chamber—The four cardiac chambers and the inferoseptal and anterolateral walls of the left ventricle can be assessed, as can be the mitral and tricuspid valves. Assess right ventricular size.

6. MO mitral commissural—Parts of both the anterior and posterior mitral valve leaflets can be seen, as well as the chordal attachments to both papillary muscles.

7. MO 2-chamber—Anterior (right screen) and inferior (left screen) LV wall. All parts of the anterior mitral valve leaflet and left atrial appendage can be seen.

8. MO LAX—Aortic valve, and anteroseptal and inferolateral LV walls (left screen).

9. MO asc. aortic SAX—Main pulmonary artery and right pulmonary artery; left pulmonary artery not well visualised. Useful for assessing the position of the tip of a pulmonary artery catheter. May assist in the diagnosis of massive pulmonary embolism.

10. MO asc. aortic LAX—Ascending aorta and right pulmonary artery (top screen near transducer).

11. MO desc. aortic SAX—Assessment of atheroma; left pleural effusion may be seen.

12. UO aortic arch LAX—Aortic atheroma; aortic dissection flap.

13. UO aortic arch SAX—Useful for interrogation of the pulmonary valve; good alignment for interrogation using PW Doppler.

14. MO desc. aortic LAX—Length of the descending aorta can be seen; useful for correct positioning of the intraaortic balloon pump just distal to origin of the left subclavian artery.

15. TG basal SAX—Assessment of mitral valve pathology; origin of mitral valve regurgitant jet; mitral valve repair.

16. TG LAX—Good alignment for interrogation of aortic valve using Doppler.

17. TG mid SAX—Both papillary muscles seen; LV regions supplied by left anterior descending, left circumflex and right coronary arteries. Best view for calculating fractional area change; assessment of regional ischaemia. Right ventricular free wall to the left of screen.

18. TG 2-chamber—Mitral subvalvular apparatus; left atrial appendage.

19. TG RV inflow—Inferior wall of RV and the tricuspid valve.

20. Deep TG LAX—Good alignment for use of Doppler or CFD to assess aortic, mitral or pulmonary valves.

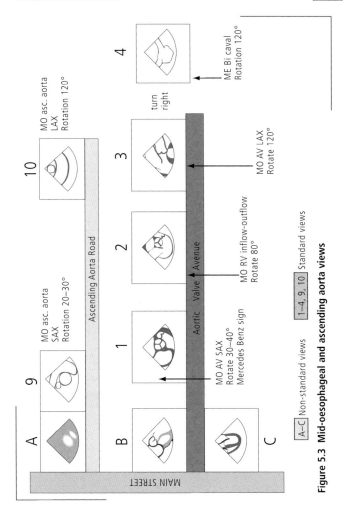

Figure 5.3 **Mid-oesophageal and ascending aorta views**

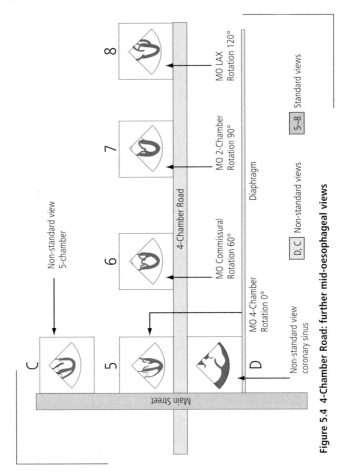

Figure 5.4 4-Chamber Road: further mid-oesophageal views

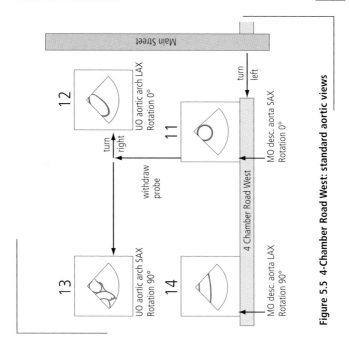

Figure 5.5 4-Chamber Road West: standard aortic views

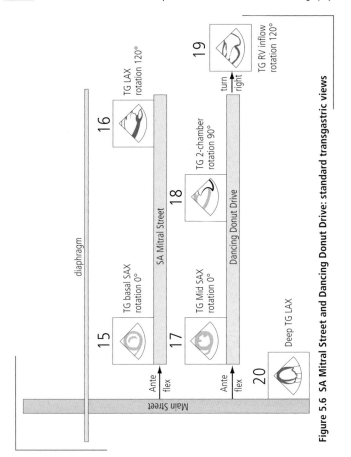

Figure 5.6 SA Mitral Street and Dancing Donut Drive: standard transgastric views

Chapter 6

Standard transthoracic echocardiography examination

Michael Veltman and John Faris

Learning objectives

1. Learn the windows that are used for TTE.
2. Identify the structures seen in the basic windows using 2D, and 2D plus CFD.
3. Identify the imaging views for commonly used spectral Doppler imaging for TTE.
4. Understand how to conduct the standard TTE examination.

Positioning the patient

Positioning the patient correctly will help considerably in obtaining good quality images, but is not always possible in the critical care environment. It is possible to image from either the left or right side of the patient, but the following instructions will assume that the operator is located on the left side and therefore will be holding the probe in the left hand while operating the controls with the right hand. The best results will be obtained when the environment is dark and quiet.

The optimal patient position for the parasternal and apical windows is generally left lateral decubitus, with the patient's head lying on the left hand, which will roll the heart forward on to the chest wall close to the probe.

The basic windows

The subcostal and suprasternal windows available for TTE are defined predominantly by the bony structures of the chest wall (i.e. the sternum, clavicles and ribs), because these are barriers to ultrasound transmission. The anterior chest wall, which has multiple rib inter-spaces where imaging is possible, is divided into the apical and parasternal windows, and their exact location will vary according to individual anatomy (e.g. dilated heart in disease states), changes in posture and the degree of lung inflation. An understanding of the ideal views will allow the best positioning of the probe for each individual.

The parasternal window

The parasternal window allows assessment of the long and short axes of the heart. Long-axis views should be obtained first by placing the probe in the 4th rib interspace as close to the sternum as possible with the index marker pointing towards the patient's right shoulder. If the image quality is poor, moving up or down an interspace or slightly towards the apex may bring the chambers into view. A depth of around 14 cm is usually sufficient to see all the structures.

 Parasternal long axis: The long-axis view allows assessment of the left heart in detail, during M-mode (for aorta/atrial size and LV dimensions), zooming in on areas of interest such as the mitral and aortic valves, and performing CFD of the valves.

 Parasternal right ventricular inflow: Angulation of the probe in this plane towards the right upper quadrant of the abdomen will produce a view of the RV inflow in which the tricuspid valve can be seen and regurgitation assessed with CFD and PW Doppler.

Parasternal right ventricular outflow: Angulation in the oppo-site direction (towards the left shoulder) may produce a view of the RV outflow tract in some individuals, enabling assessment of the PV.

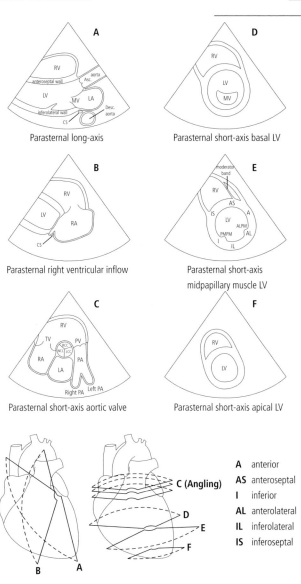

Parasternal long-axis

Parasternal short-axis basal LV

Parasternal right ventricular inflow

Parasternal short-axis
midpapillary muscle LV

Parasternal short-axis aortic valve

Parasternal short-axis apical LV

A   anterior
AS anteroseptal
I   inferior
AL anterolateral
IL inferolateral
IS inferoseptal

Figure 6.1 Parasternal window

Parasternal short axis (apical, mid, basal): To change from the parasternal long-axis to the short-axis view the transducer is rotated clockwise on the skin without other movement until the index marker points to the left shoulder. From here angulation can identify the ventricle in multiple planes by changing the angle of the probe—without changing the point at which the probe touches the patient if possible. Angulation towards the apex of the heart produces an apical short-axis view, and changing the angle from there slowly towards the right shoulder will then produce a mid-papillary view of the LV, in which the two papillary muscles are visible. (The apical cut has no objects seen in the left ventricular cavity.)

Further angulation of the probe towards the right shoulder will produce a basal window (with the MV seen in cross-section as a 'fish-mouth').

These three short-axis views allow assessment of LV wall motion using the standard 17-segment model (see Chapter 4). The basal short-axis view also allows assessment of the MV using CFD.

Parasternal short axis (aortic valve): Continuing to angle the probe towards the right shoulder will bring into view the aortic valve in the short axis. Further angulation beyond this in some subjects can produce a short-axis view of the ascending aorta above the aortic valve.

This is an excellent view for assessing the TV and PV using 2D, CFD and spectral Doppler. The aortic valve is also seen in short axis, enabling 2D and CFD assessment. The RV free wall is seen at the top of the sector. Occasionally this view will also reveal abnormalities in the atrial septum or more distal pulmonary trunk.

The apical window

The apical window is located (not surprisingly) close to the apex of the LV. The exact location varies but is generally close to where the apex beat can be felt. The probe is held with the index marker point-ing to the patient's left side, with a sector depth of approximately 18 cm.

Apical 4-chamber: The initial view should be the apical 4-chamber view. The inferoseptal (septal) and anterolateral (lateral) of the LV are seen, as well as its true apex. The free wall of the RV is also seen. Assessment of the MV and TV is performed using 2D, CFD and

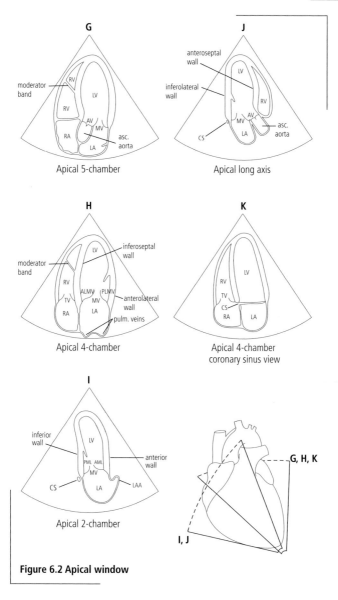

G Apical 5-chamber

moderator band
RV
RV
LV
AV
MV
RA
LA
asc. aorta

J Apical long axis

anteroseptal wall
inferolateral wall
LV
RV
AV
MV
CS
LA
asc. aorta

H Apical 4-chamber

moderator band
inferoseptal wall
LV
RV
ALMV PLMV
TV
MV
RA
LA
anterolateral wall
pulm. veins

K Apical 4-chamber coronary sinus view

LV
RV
TV
CS
RA
LA

I Apical 2-chamber

inferior wall
LV
PML AML
MV
CS
LA
anterior wall
LAA

G, H, K

I, J

Figure 6.2 Apical window

spectral Doppler of mitral (and sometimes tricuspid) inflow, plus interrogation of tricuspid or mitral regurgitant jets. Additional measurements of the pulmonary vein flow velocities and tissue Doppler of the mitral annulus can be performed.

Apical 5-chamber: Angulation of the probe towards the patient's head will produce a 5-chamber view, and a 4-chamber coronary sinus view if angled towards the abdomen. The 5-chamber view in particular enables assessment of flow velocities in the LVOT and through the aortic valve; in addition to CFD assessment of aortic regurgitation. This is one of the best views for obtaining Doppler measurements to calculate cardiac output.

Apical 2-chamber: Rotation of the probe in the apical window from the 4-chamber view counter clockwise will produce a 2-chamber window (at approximately 90° from the 4-chamber view with the probe index marker pointing towards the patient's head). It should be noted that the probe angle in the 2-chamber view is perpendicular to the rib interspaces, which makes it one of the harder views to obtain. The anterior and inferior walls of the LV are seen in this view, as is the MV, which can be assessed using 2D and CFD (there is usually no benefit in repeating flow velocities from the 4-chamber view).

Apical long axis: An apical long-axis view is seen at approximately 120° counter clockwise rotation from the original 4-chamber view. Typically, the index marker is pointing towards the patient's right shoulder. Assessment of the anteroseptal and posterolateral (posterior) walls of the LV can be made using 2D. Additional views of the MV and AV can be obtained with 2D and CFM. This is a good window for repeating measurements of aortic valve gradients if aortic stenosis is suspected from the 2D images.

The subcostal window

The subcostal window is located below the ribs, and the best probe position is either to the left or right of the midline. The optimal position for most patients while the subcostal window is viewed is supine. Cooperative patients can be asked to bend their knees up, which will usually enable a better view of the heart to be obtained. This window is further away from the heart than the apical or parasternal windows and a sector depth of 20–24 cm is commonly required in an adult.

Subcostal 4-chamber: With the index marker pointing to the patient's left side, the subcostal 4-chamber view can be seen, in which the MV and TV can be assessed using 2D and CFD; however, generally the angle is poor for Doppler measurements. The subcostal window is usually the best for detecting atrial (and sometimes ventricular) septal defects using CFD.

Subcostal short axis: Rotation of the probe by approximately 90° will produce a short-axis view of the heart, similar to the parasternal window; angulation of the probe will potentially enable views from the apex to the base of the heart. Apical views may be hard to obtain, but the mid-papillary short axis up to the AV short axis can be easily found in most subjects.

Subcostal IVC: Further angulation towards the patient's right will produce a view of the IVC as it enters the right atrium. The size of the vessel and the degree of collapse during spontaneous ventilation is used to assess right atrial pressure.

Subcostal descending aorta: Orientation of the transducer plane to the vertical and aiming towards the descending aorta will produce a view between the above with the aorta in long axis.

The suprasternal window

The suprasternal window is a difficult plane and may not be possible in all subjects. It does, however, enable visualisation of the aorta from ascending through the arch to the initial descending thoracic aorta. The aortic valve can sometimes be seen, and may be assessed using CW Doppler (even when not visualised) as an additional assessment of aortic valve gradients. CFD and PW Doppler of the arch and descending aorta enables assessment of coarctation of the aorta, and very occasionally dissection may be seen on 2D imaging.

The standard examination

A complete standard examination requires a basic knowledge of the four windows: parasternal, apical, subcostal and suprasternal. Within each of these windows, several planes can be seen by varying the angulation and rotation of the probe. The windows have been

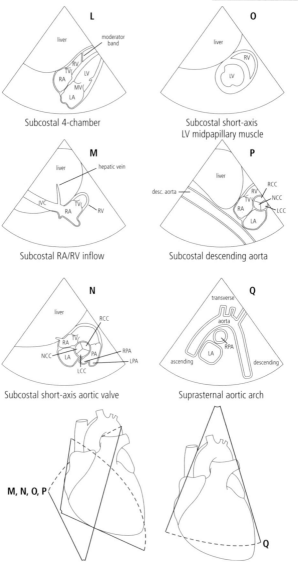

Subcostal 4-chamber

Subcostal short-axis
LV midpapillary muscle

Subcostal RA/RV inflow

Subcostal descending aorta

Subcostal short-axis aortic valve

Suprasternal aortic arch

Figure 6.3 Subcostal and suprasternal windows

standardised into several views, all of which should be sought. Within each view all structures should be reviewed in 2D, and where appropriate, interrogated with M-mode, CFD and spectral Doppler.

Suggested order

Parasternal

1. Long axis (LV function, aortic/atrial size, MV, AV)
2. RV inflow (TV structure and function, TV regurgitant jet gradient, RV function)
3. Aortic valve short axis (TV, PV, AV)
4. Basal, mid and apical short axis (LV segmental function)

Apical

5. 4-chamber (mitral/pulmonary vein flow, LV function: inferoseptal (septal)/anterolateral (lateral), TV)
6. 5-chamber (LVOT and AV spectral and CFD)
7. 2-chamber (LV function: anterior/inferior walls; MV)
8. long axis (LV function: anteroseptal/inferolateral (posterior) walls; MV, AV)

Subcostal

9. 4-chamber (atrial and ventricular septum, LV function, MV, TV)
10. Mid and basal short axis (LV function)
11. Aortic valve short axis (TV, PV structure and flow, AV)
12. IVC (collapse and flow reversal)
13. Descending aorta

Suprasternal

14. Aorta long axis (AV, aortic dissection and coarctation)

Writing the report

Because the TTE examination can produce an enormous amount of information about cardiac structure and function, a systematic approach is strongly recommended so that nothing is overlooked. Time may not permit this in the critically ill patient, but if a limited examination is performed then any views that have been omitted should be documented.

Because the assessment is based on views rather than structures, a worksheet on which to record the findings during the examination is valuable, particularly if the echocardiography machine does not record the measurements.

To make the report concise, a suggested order for documenting the findings is given. Measurements can be stated either at the start of the report or included in the text. A summary of the major findings (and any recommendations) should comprise the conclusion.

Order of the report

1. Left ventricular size and function (diastolic function assessment)
2. Right ventricular size and function
3. Atria
4. Mitral valve
5. Aortic valve
6. Pulmonary and tricuspid valves
7. Pericardium and aorta
8. Conclusion

Chapter 7

Introduction to Doppler imaging and equations

Colin Iatrou

Learning objectives
1. Understand Doppler imaging, including pulsed wave, continuous wave and colour flow.
2. Perform a Doppler examination using basic Doppler measurements.
3. Use Doppler measurements, the Bernoulli equation and continuity principle for basic calculations, including cardiac output, valve area and right ventricular systolic pressure.

Understanding Doppler imaging

All the measurements and calculations discussed in this chapter are based on a fundamental principle known as the Doppler effect, named after Austrian physicist Christian Johann Doppler (1805–1853) who observed that the pitch of sound heard by a stationary observer varied with the speed of the emitting object. The Doppler effect is well demonstrated by the example of a speeding emergency vehicle (Figure 7.1). When the vehicle moves towards the stationary observer, the pitch (or frequency, f) of the siren is higher than when the vehicle speeds away. When the vehicle is stationary the pitch is constant. The change in

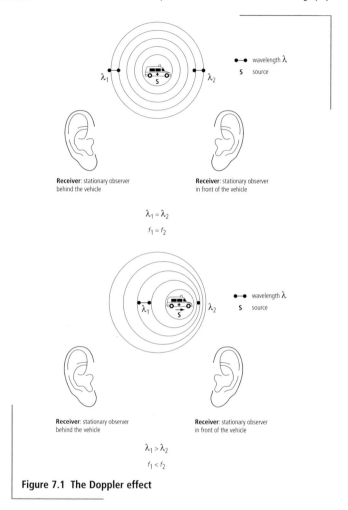

$$\lambda_1 = \lambda_2$$
$$f_1 = f_2$$

$$\lambda_1 > \lambda_2$$
$$f_1 < f_2$$

Figure 7.1 The Doppler effect

frequency of the moving vehicle compared with the stationary vehicle is called the Doppler shift and is caused by the compression of sound waves in front (decreased wavelength, λ), and rarefaction of the sound waves behind the vehicle (increased wavelength).

The change in frequency (Δf) or Doppler shift is described by the simple equation:

$$\Delta f = f_r - f_t$$

where f_r is the frequency of the reflected wave and f_t is the frequency of the transmitted (or incident) wave.

In echocardiography this phenomenon occurs when an ultrasound wave is reflected back to a stationary transducer by a moving red blood cell. As the cell moves towards the transducer the reflected wave has a higher frequency than the transmitted wave (positive Δf), and as the red blood cell moves away, the frequency of the reflected wave is less than that of the transmitted wave (negative Δf).

The Doppler instrument can calculate the velocity of the red cell (or quantum of red cells caught by the incident beam) using the Doppler equation:

$$\Delta f = \frac{2 f_t \, v \, \cos\theta}{c}$$

where v is the velocity of the red cells, f_t is the transmitted (incident) frequency, c is the speed of sound in soft tissue or blood (a constant, 1540 m/s), θ is the angle of incidence of the beam with the flow of blood, and doubling the value (i.e. × 2) takes into account the 'double' Doppler shift that occurs (a) when the transducer (source) emits an echo that hits a reflector (the receiver) and (b) when a returning echo produced by the reflector (source) is received by the transducer.

If the Doppler beam is aligned with the flow of blood (i.e. $\theta = 0$), then $\cos\theta = 1$, and rearranging the equation leaves a very simple calculation for the velocity of the red cell sample volume:

$$v = \frac{\Delta f c}{2 f_t}$$

which leads to an important point. The machine assumes a θ value of 0°, so if the ultrasound beam is not in line with the blood flow, an error is introduced. This raises the question 'What is acceptable alignment?' The answer lies in the relationship between θ and $\cos\theta$. If the angle of the beam is within 20° then $\cos 20 = 0.94$ and the error (or underestimation) is 7%. However, once the angle reaches 30° then $\cos 30 = 0.87$ or underestimation of 13%. Hence the accepted incident transducer angle is less than 20° (Figure 7.2).

The spectral display is the form in which the measured Doppler velocities are represented on the screen (Figure 7.3). It is a graphical display of time on the x-axis and velocity on the y-axis. An ultrasound

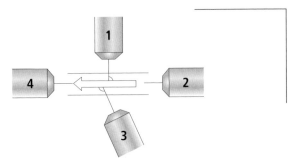

1 Transducer is interrogating flow at 90°: there will be no Doppler shift and therefore, no flow detected.

2 Transducer is interrogating at angles parallel to the flow: maximal (optimal) Doppler shift and therefore velocity will be derived. The flow profile will be negative (below baseline) because the flow is AWAY from the transducer.

3 Transducer is interrogating the flow at an angle. An incident angle of less than 20° is acceptable, greater than that and the velocity will be UNDERESTIMATED.

4 Transducer is interrogating at angles parallel to the flow: maximal (optimal) Doppler shift and therefore velocity will be derived. The flow profile will be positive (above baseline) because the flow is TOWARDS the transducer.

Figure 7.2 Effect of incident angle on perceived velocity

wave is emitted by the transducer, then received and processed by the same transducer calculating the Doppler shift, which is converted to a velocity. The brightness of the signal reflects the number of red cells travelling at that velocity. The y-axis denotes velocity and the sign (+ or −) denotes the direction of flow. Positive (flow displayed above the baseline) indicates flow towards the transducer and negative (flow displayed below the baseline) is flow away from the transducer. The x-axis reflects the timing of the signal.

Pulsed wave Doppler enables sampling of the velocity at a specific depth from the transducer. The ultrasound signal is transmitted from the transducer and is allowed to return before a further signal is emitted. As the speed of the wave in tissue is assumed to be a constant 1540 m/s, the time taken for the return signal is directly proportional to the distance from the transducer (Figure 7.4). The distance calculation is:

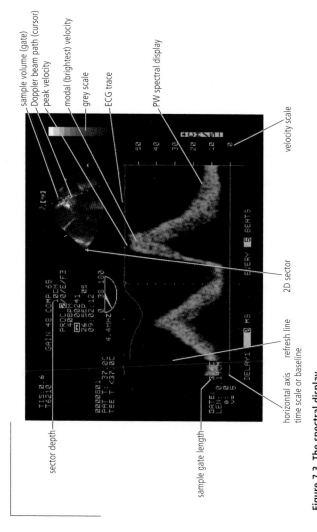

Figure 7.3 The spectral display

$$s = \frac{ct}{2}$$

where s is the distance of the reflector from the transducer, c is the speed of sound and t is the time from pulse emission to reception, and the result is halved because it is a 'round trip' (transducer to reflector to transducer).

Hence, the distance can be controlled by the operator by placing the sample volume in the area of interest, which effectively sets the 'waiting period' of the transducer. The 'waiting period' limits the number of times the transducer can cycle per second; the cycle is called the pulse repetition frequency (PRF). In theory, if the sample to be interrogated is close to the transducer, the PRF will be high, and it will be low if the sample volume is at a greater depth. In fact, in order to get an unambiguous measure of the direction of a Doppler shift, each returning wave must be interrogated at least twice in its cycle.

This is often compared to a motion picture of a rotating wagon wheel (Figure 7.5). If the frame rate of the film reel is greater than twice the rotation of the wheel, the wagon will be seen to go forward. If the wheel speeds up so that the frame rate is less than twice the wheel rotation, it will seem to go backwards. This is known as frequency aliasing and the frequency at which aliasing occurs is known as the Nyquist limit (i.e. half the pulse repetition frequency). On the spectral display, the part of the signal that is beyond the Nyquist limit appears as a 'cut off' of the signal in one channel and the appearance of the amputated part in the reverse channel (Figure 7.6a, b). This is known as signal aliasing and occurs because the transducer cannot unambiguously assign direction to the Doppler shift.

One method of overcoming aliasing is to use continuous wave

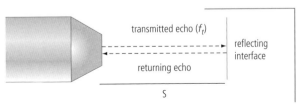

Figure 7.4 Distance calculation

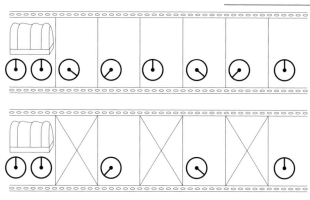

Figure 7.5 Frequency aliasing analogy

Doppler. When interrogating in CW mode the transducer acts as a continuous transmitter and receiver. Because the sampling frequency is continuous, very high frequency shifts (velocities: >2 m/s) can be measured, such as aortic stenosis jets. The disadvantage is there is no 'waiting time', so there is a lack of depth perception (i.e. the depth of the sample cannot be determined). Reflected velocities from samples all along the sampling line are displayed and it is the operator's task to deduce where the peak velocity sample is by placing the interrogation line (cursor) through the flow disturbance to be measured. In Figure 7.7, for example, the CW cursor is aimed through the aortic valve. Notice that CW has a spectral wave area that is 'filled in' compared with PW, because the full range of frequencies is represented by multiple samples along the entire length of the scan line.

Colour flow Doppler is a form of PW that uses multiple interrogations along a line, and sequentially on adjacent lines, to create a window or sector of colour flow over the 2D image (Figure 7.8). Each sample in the scan line is analysed for Doppler shift and assigned a colour representing velocity and direction. By convention, flow towards the transducer is designated a shade of red, and flow away is designated a shade of blue. The shade is correlated with a shade scale shown on the side of the display. If, despite scale and gain adjustment, the Nyquist limit is exceeded, then a mosaic of colour is shown, which indicates turbulent flow. Thus CFD is a useful semi-quantitative mapping tool for assessing blood flow.

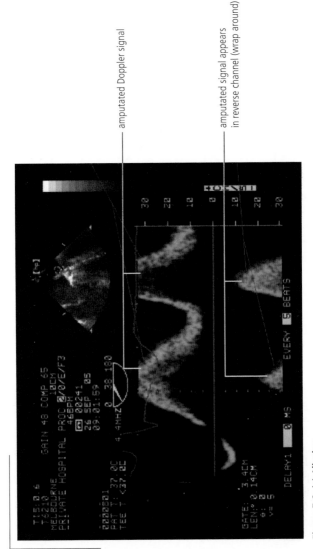

Figure 7.6 (a) Aliasing

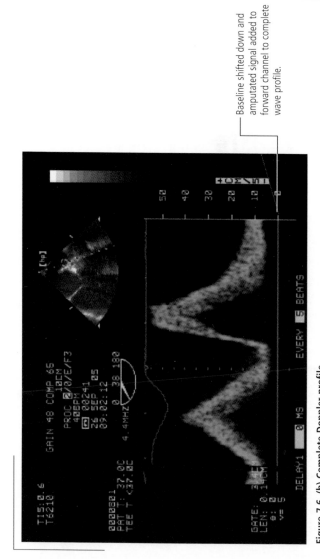

Baseline shifted down and amputated signal added to forward channel to complete wave profile.

Figure 7.6 (b) Complete Doppler profile

CW cursor

AV

Measurements and calculations
performed by the machine software.
Note maximum velocity, velocity time integral (VTI)
mean pressure gradient
and maximum pressure gradient

CW Doppler signal
Notice the wave is 'filled in' because
of the wide range of velocities along
the line of interrogation

Doppler profile traced by operator

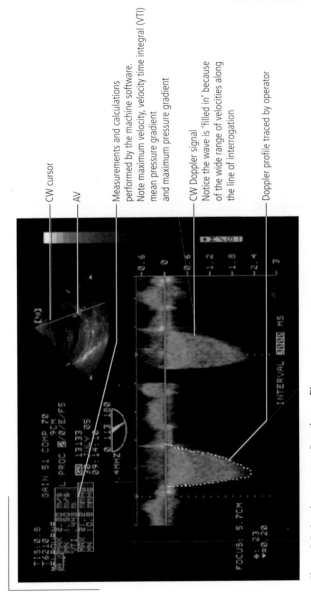

Figure 7.7 Continuous wave Doppler profile

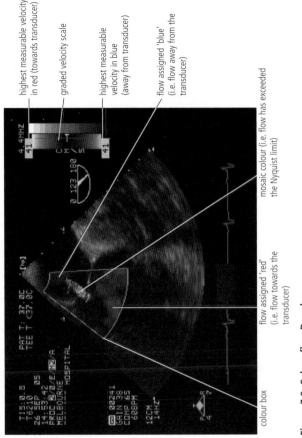

highest measurable velocity in red (towards transducer)

graded velocity scale

highest measurable velocity in blue (away from transducer)

flow assigned 'blue' (i.e. flow away from the transducer)

mosaic colour (i.e. flow has exceeded the Nyquist limit)

flow assigned 'red' (i.e. flow towards the transducer)

colour box

Figure 7.8 Colour flow Doppler

The standard Doppler examination

Armed with a basic understanding of Doppler ultrasound, it becomes a simple task to direct the ultrasound beam through the area to be examined. With PW and CW, the line of interrogation must be directed to within 20° of the direction of flow. When using PW, the sample volume must also be set to the required depth using the cursor control. If there is signal aliasing, the velocity scale of the display may be increased, which increases the PRF and the maximum measurable frequency shift. Also, the operator can perform an electronic 'cut and paste' by shifting the baseline on the spectral display up or down. The 'amputated' signal from the reverse channel is now added to the forward channel to complete the signal (Figure 7.6b). If aliasing still occurs, then CW must be used. It is assumed that the highest velocity on the display is returning from the sample of interest (e.g. stenotic valve) as very few samples on the one line would achieve velocities of this magnitude (Figure 7.7). However, the operator should be familiar with the 'typical' Doppler profiles and the timing in the cardiac cycle of the flows being interrogated, which is of particular importance when there are co-existing valvular pathologies.

The position and width of a colour flow sector can usually be set using the trackball. The 2D image combined with CFD can give vital information on the velocity, direction, length, and overall pattern of the blood flow or jet. It is recommended that the sector is the minimum width and length necessary to obtain the desired information because it will help to maintain a suitable frame rate. If the colour sector is too large, it will reduce the frame rate causing the real-time image to appear 'sluggish', consistent with poor temporal resolution. Instrument settings will affect the apparent size and magnitude of the jet. Colour gain should be increased until speckling appears in the soft tissues, then turned down slightly until the speckling just disappears. The velocity scale should be increased enough to prevent aliasing of the signal. For low-velocity jets it may be necessary to lower the scale. These techniques are part of a process called 'image optimisation'.

Measurements on the spectral display should always be made on a frozen image. Most machines provide a caliper and a trace function. When measuring velocity through the pulmonary or aortic valves, the highest velocity in the range (outer edge) should be traced, whereas with the atrioventricular valves, the modal (brightest) velocity should be traced (Figure 7.7).

The Bernoulli equation

The Bernoulli equation is based on the law of the conservation of energy and relates the pressure drop along a tube to the velocity of the fluid in that tube. It is used to convert velocity to pressure; that is, pressure change = convective acceleration + flow acceleration + viscous friction:

$$\Delta P = 1/2\rho\,(V_2{}^2 - V_1{}^2) + \int_1^2 dV/dt \times ds + R(V)$$

where ρ is the density of fluid, V_1 is the proximal velocity, V_2 is the distal velocity, dV/dt is the change of velocity over time, ds is the distance over which the pressure changes, R is the viscous resistance in the vessel and V is the velocity of flow (m/s).

A simplified/modified Bernoulli equation is derived from making the following assumptions: (1) acceleration is zero at peak velocities, (2) viscous friction is ignored because the flow interrogated in the centre of a vessel lumen is usually flat, (3) mass density in normal blood is four, and (4) there is conservation of energy.

$$\Delta P = 4(V_2{}^2 - V_1{}^2)$$

V_1 is usually insignificant and, if less than 1.2 m/s, may be ignored and the following equation is routinely used:

$$\Delta P = 4V^2$$

where ΔP is the pressure gradient in mmHg and V is the velocity of the jet (m/s).

When a wave is traced from baseline to baseline, peak velocity, mean velocity, peak pressure gradient, mean pressure gradient and velocity–time integral (VTI) are usually indicated on the screen.

Peak velocity (m/s): The operator can use the machine calculations package or a simple generic caliper placed at the maximum point (velocity) of the spectral Doppler display generated from the flow of interest (Figure 7.9).

Mean velocity (m/s): The machine software derives this parameter by averaging many points in the spectral trace (Figure 7.10).

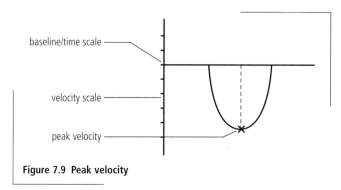

Figure 7.9 Peak velocity

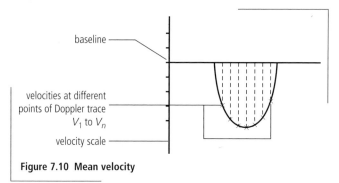

Figure 7.10 Mean velocity

Peak pressure gradient (mmHg): The peak pressure gradient is manually calculated by the operator or automatically generated by the machine software using the peak velocity of the flow being interrogated and applying the modified/simplified Bernoulli equation (Figure 7.9).

Mean pressure gradient (mmHg): The mean pressure gradient is a parameter calculated by the machine software once the operator has traced the spectral Doppler profile. The machine derives this measurement by measuring many velocities (V_n) at regular intervals on the spectral Doppler trace (Figure 7.10) and applying the modified Bernoulli equation.

$$\text{Mean pressure gradient} = \frac{4V_1^2 + 4V_2^2 + 4V_3^2 + 4V_4^2 + 4V_5^2 \ldots + 4V_n^2}{n}$$

Velocity–time integral (cm):   The area under the velocity–time curve. It is the entire volume of flow in a given ejection period. It is calculated by the machine software once the operator has selected 'VTI' in the calculations package and traced around the spectral Doppler waveform. It is used preferentially to peak velocity in continuity equation applications because it eliminates some of the error that may arise by not being in the exact location where the diameter for cross-sectional area (CSA) has been measured.

Right ventricular systolic pressure: Pressure gradient determinations are valuable in diagnosing stenotic valves (Figure 7.7), but also can be used to estimate heart chamber pressures. RVSP can be estimated from the tricuspid regurgitant (TR) jet, if it is present (Figure 7.11). Because TR occurs during systole, the ΔP measured across the TV gives the pressure difference between the right ventricle and atrium: RVSP = $4(V_{TR})^2$ + RAP.

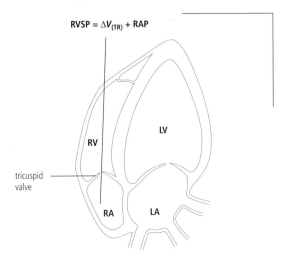

$$RVSP = \Delta V_{(TR)} + RAP$$

Transthoracic apical 4-chamber
CW cursor through the TV leaflets interrogating the TR jet (if present) in systole.

Figure 7.11 TTE view for measuring RVSP

Estimating right atrial pressure

Right atrial pressure (RAP) is presumed to be 10–15 mmHg if the jugular venous pressure (JVP) is normal or 20 mmHg if the JVP is elevated. It can be directly measured if a right atrial catheter has been inserted.

Alternatively RAP can be estimated by assessing the size and motion 'collapsibility' of the IVC in the TTE subcostal view (Table 7.1), either by direct visualisation or by placing the M-mode cursor through the IVC and using generic calipers to measure the IVC at the largest diameter (during expiration) and smallest diameter (during inspiration, aided by asking the patient to 'sniff').

Table 7.1 Estimation of right atrial pressure

IVC size (cm)	IVC collapse with inspiration	Estimated RAP (mmHg)	Grade of RAP
<1.5	>50%	0–5	Low
1.5–2.5	>50%	5–10	Normal
1.5–2.5	<50%	10–15	Mild elevation
>2.5	<50%	15–20	Moderate elevation
>2.5 (dilated)	Fixed/no collapse	>20	Severe elevation

Calculating cardiac output and area of valves

Measurement of cardiac output (CO) is a simple and valuable application of Doppler imaging. If it is imagined that each heart beat results in the ejection of a cylindrical column of blood into the aorta, then the integral of the velocity–time waveform can be thought of as the height of this column or the average distance a blood cell travels in one beat (Figure 7.12). Multiplying this by the cross-sectional area (CSA) of the left ventricular outflow tract (LVOT) will give the volume of the cylinder or the stroke volume (SV), which can then be multiplied by heart rate (HR) to give CO:

$$CO = HR \times SV \text{ or}$$
$$CO = HR \times (CSA \times VTI)$$

The CSA can be calculated using basic trigonometry. The diameter (*D*) in centimetres of the LVOT is measured on 2D ultrasound and substituted in the formula:

$$\text{CSA} = \pi(D/2)^2$$

Note that this calculation works anywhere in the heart that both VTI and CSA can be measured accurately, however, it seems to be simplest and most convenient at the LVOT.

The continuity principle is based on the law of conservation of mass, which when applied to fluid systems states that, provided there is no loss of fluid from the system, whatever flows in, must flow out. This law is used extensively in echocardiography to measure valve areas, regurgitant areas and regurgitant volumes, as well as shunt fractions. The continuity principle applies to the AV; that is, for a given heartbeat, the flow through the LVOT is equal to the flow through the valve. Because SV is a constant, thus:

$$\text{SV}_{(AV)} = \text{SV}_{(LVOT)}$$

$$\text{CSA}_{(AV)} \times \text{VTI}_{(AV)} = \text{CSA}_{(LVOT)} \times \text{VTI}_{(LVOT)}$$

Rearranging the equation:

$$\text{CSA(AV)} = \frac{\text{CSA}_{(LVOT)} \times \text{VTI}_{(LVOT)}}{\text{VTI}_{(AV)}}$$

the CSA of the AV can be calculated.

Note that in order to obtain $\text{VTI}_{(LVOT)}$, PW Doppler must be used with the cursor sample placed below the AV in the LVOT. To measure the $\text{VTI}_{(AV)}$, CW Doppler is aimed through the AV (Figure 7.13). As the highest velocity on the CW line of interrogation is at the AV, the peak velocity envelope will be reflected from there (Figure 7.13). It is recommended that the VTI is measured and averaged for at least 3–5 beats in sinus rhythm and 8–10 beats in arrhythmia such as atrial fibrillation. The operator must also be aware that the presence of an intracardiac shunt (membranous ventricular septal defect) may render inaccurate the calculation of the AV area by the continuity equation.

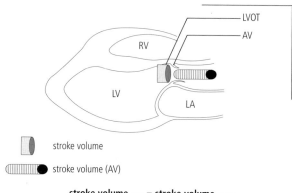

Figure 7.12 Continuity principle

Summary of the equations

Bernoulli equation
$$\Delta P = 1/2\rho\,(V_2^2 - V_1^2) + \int_1^2 dV/dt \times ds + R(V)$$

Modified/simplified Bernoulli equation
$$\Delta P = 4(V_2^2 - V_1^2) \text{ or}$$

$$\Delta P = 4V^2 \text{ (when } V_1 <1.2 \text{ m/s)}$$

Cross-sectional area
$$CSA = \pi(D/2)^2$$

Stroke volume
$$SV = CSA \times VTI$$

Heart rate (beats/min)
$$HR = (R \text{ to } R \text{ interval}) \times 60$$

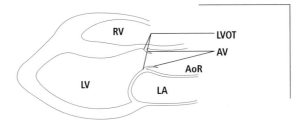

Transthoracic parasternal long axis

LVOT diameter is taken at mid systole when the AV leaflets are open at their maximum. Measure 'inner edge to inner edge' at leaflet insertion.

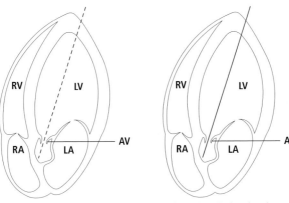

Transthoracic apical 5-chamber

PW Doppler is activated with the sample gate at the LVOT (either at the AV annulus or within 0.5–1.0 cm proximal to it on the LV side)

Transthoracic apical 5-chamber

CW Doppler is activated, interrogating the AV (for aortic valve area)

Figure 7.13 TTE views for obtaining parameters for the continuity equation (CO or AV area)

Cardiac output (L/min)

$$CO = HR \times SV \text{ or}$$
$$CO = HR \times (CSA \times VTI)$$

Cardiac index (L/min per m^2)

$$CI = \frac{CO}{BSA}$$

Continuity equation

$$CSA_1 \times VTI_1 = CSA_2 \times VTI_2$$

$$CSA_2 = \frac{CSA_1 \times VTI_1}{VTI_2}$$

$$\text{Example: AV area} = \frac{CSA_{(LVOT)} \times VTI_{(LVOT)}}{VTI_{(AV)}}$$

RVSP

Using TR: $RVSP = 4(V_{TR})^2 + RAP$

(Note: PAP = RVSP in the absence of RVOT obstruction)

Chapter 8

Assessing the basic haemodynamic state

Colin Royse

Learning objectives

1. Know the 7 basic haemodynamic states.
2. Know the 4 steps of the basic haemodynamic assessment.
3. Understand how diagnosis of the haemodynamic state can assist patient management

The basic haemodynamic states

This chapter introduces the concept of the haemodynamic state and its evaluation using different facets of the information obtained from the echocardiography examination to rapidly determine which of the seven basic haemodynamic states the patient is in. The ways in which the haemodynamic evaluation helps clinical management are also discussed.

The method of assessment will vary between TOE and TTE, but the basic premise is understanding how to assess the patient's haemodynamic state. The transthoracic assessment can become very complex, so for the purpose of this chapter the information has been kept relatively simple.

The seven haemodynamic states

In patient management, cardiovascular parameters are broadly cate-gorised as normal or abnormal. The first of the seven basic haemo-dynamic states is 'normal', in which there are no abnormalities of blood pressure, heart rate or general body functioning, including urine output and acid–base homeostasis. With invasive haemody-namic monitoring, a right atrial pressure or pulmonary capillary wedge pressure (PCWP) of less than 15 mmHg and a cardiac index (CI) greater than 2.5 L/min per m^2 would be taken as indicators of normal cardiovascular status.

The most commonly detected haemodynamic abnormality is a fall in blood pressure (hypotension), which is readily detectable with non-invasive or invasive monitoring. Other features of an abnormal haemodynamic state would include a fall in urine output, poor tissue perfusion, increasing acidosis, reduced cardiac output, and high or low filling pressures. Although these signs indicate an abnormal haemodynamic state, it is not necessarily easy to categorise the cause without using imaging technology such as echocardiography. A low CI in association with a high PCWP, for example, could be caused by a dilated, poorly contracting LV, or by a small stiff ventricle as seen with severe diastolic dysfunction. It is important to appreciate that there may be hybrids of the basic haemodynamic states; for example, a failing LV could also be subjected to excessive vasodilation in the presence of a systemic inflammatory response syndrome.

The seven basic haemodynamic states are as follows:
- Normal
- Empty (hypovolaemia)
- Primary diastolic failure
- Primary systolic failure
- Systolic and diastolic failure
- Vasodilation
- Right ventricular failure.

The basic haemodynamic assessment

There are four steps to the basic haemodynamic assessment, whether it is conducted during TOE or TTE:
1. Estimate volume
2. Estimate systolic function

3. Estimate filling pressure
4. Final assessment (putting it all together).

Step 1. Estimate volume (preload)

Prior to the introduction of non-invasive monitoring with echocardiography, LV volume was inferred from measuring the right atrial pressure (RAP) or the PCWP. As a general rule, as either RAP or PCWP increased, so did the end-diastolic volume (EDV). What could not be determined from invasive pressure monitoring, however, was the compliance of the LV. A PCWP of 18 mmHg could occur in a patient with a dilated LV, and equally could occur in one with an underfilled LV and severe diastolic dysfunction. With echocardiography, LV volume can be directly estimated by one of several methods.

M-mode echocardiography: A one-dimensional estimation of preload is possible in this mode. Traditionally, in TOE the cursor is directed through the base of the LV at the level of the tips of the MV from the TG basal view or from the TG 90° view. When using TTE, the M-mode is obtained from a parasternal long- or short-axis view through the base of the LV and the end-diastolic dimension (LVEDD) is measured at the point of the Q-wave on the ECG. The range of 'normal' values will vary between laboratories and across populations, but a 'working range' is 4.0–5.5 cm. It is recommended to index the LVEDD to the patient's BSA and the normal indexed range is 2.3–3.1 cm/m². If the LVEDD exceeds 5.4 cm, then the ventricle is dilated, and if it is less than 2.3 cm it is in a hypovolaemic state. There are several formulae for converting the single dimension into a volume, such as the Teichholz formula, but translating the value is not a practical help to determining the preload. Clearly, errors will be induced when using a one-dimensional measurement to determine a 3D structure, particularly when there is a significant wall motion abnormality in the base, because preload will be overestimated.

Simpson's method: This calculation method is available on most echocardiography machines, and divides the 2D image of the ventricle into a series of segments and then calculates a volume based on assumptions about the geometry of the ventricle. Although there is reasonable estimation between Simpson's method and other methods of volume assessment for TTE, there is much greater potential for error when using TOE because of the risk of foreshortening the LV in the mid-oesophageal views.

Two-dimensional imaging of the heart in the apical 4-chamber and 2-chamber views allows for the calculation of the LVEDV by the area–length and Simpson's biplane method. The endocardial border is traced at end-diastole and the ultrasound system calculates the volume/s. The normal mean LVEDV for men is 112 mL (indexed 58 mL/m^2) and for women 89 mL (indexed 50 mL/m^2).

End-diastolic area: The EDA is measured from the TG mid view, otherwise known as the 'mid-papillary view', which is familiar to most practitioners of TOE and is the view recommended for serial assessment of preload using the 'blood pool area' (Figure 8.1).

1. First obtain the TG mid view and freeze the image.
2. Scroll until the largest area is obtained (end-diastolic).
3. Trace around the endocardium of the blood pool area to obtain the left ventricular end-diastolic area (LVEDA).
4. Categorise the LVEDA as hypovolaemia (<8 cm^2), normal (8–14 cm^2) or dilated (>14 cm^2).

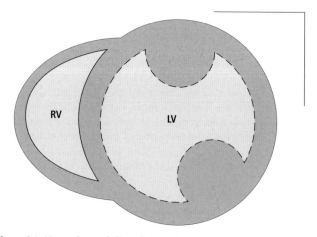

Figure 8.1 Measuring end-diastolic area (EDA) using the 'blood pool area'

Remember that preload refers to the volume status of the ventricle and is not a filling pressure. Categorise the volume based on the echocardiography examination irrespective of what the filling pressure might be.

Step 2. Estimate systolic function

For the basic haemodynamic assessment, fractional area change (FAC) derived from the TG mid view is used for TOE, and fractional shortening (FS) for TTE. After tracing the LVEDA (TOE), scroll until the smallest area is obtained (at the end of the T-wave); then trace around the blood pool area as before to determine the LV end-systolic area (LVESA). Now calculate FAC or FS using:

$$FAC = (LVEDA - LVESA)/LVEDA \text{ or}$$
$$FS = (LVEDD–LVESD)/LVEDD$$

Categorise systolic function as increased (FAC >65% or FS >44%), normal (FAC 50–65% or FS 28–44%) or reduced (FAC <50% or FS <28%) (Figure 8.3).

Step 3. Estimate filling pressure

When evaluating the basic haemodynamic state, it is important to categorise left atrial pressure (LAP) into 'high' or 'normal', and it is of some additional use to determine when the LAP might be 'low' because that can help identify a hypovolaemic state. There are many ways to estimate the LAP with echocardiography, but none of them is particularly accurate in determining the 'raw' pressure, and will always be less accurate than invasive pressure monitoring. I advise you to look at several different indices of LAP, especially if the first measurement is ambiguous. The definition of a 'high' LAP is somewhat arbitrary and is based on the years of experience with invasive pressure monitoring, such as a pulmonary artery catheter. It is probably reasonable, however, to define it as greater than 15 mmHg.

The following two methods are examples of estimating LAP and are arranged in the order of my personal preference. Other methods are beyond the scope of this book.

The shape and movement of the interatrial septum: The normal direction of the interatrial septum is from left to right for most of the cardiac cycle. During mid-systole, however, there is a transient

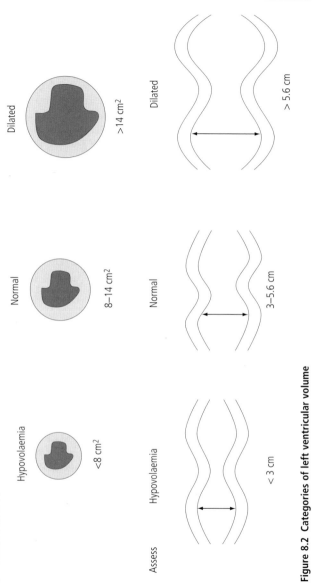

Figure 8.2 Categories of left ventricular volume

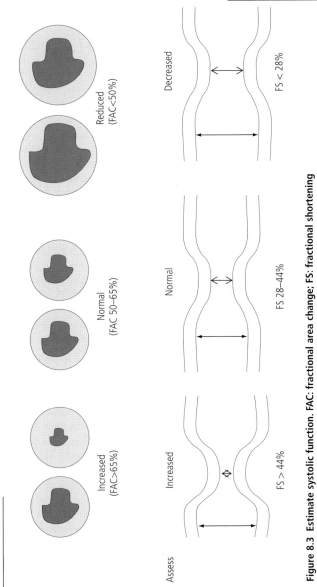

Figure 8.3 Estimate systolic function. FAC: fractional area change; FS: fractional shortening

reversal from right to left. As the LAP rises, this directional change is reduced, and when the pressure is elevated, the septum remains bowed from left to right throughout the cardiac cycle. These changes are accentuated by ventilation such that there is increased movement of the interatrial septum. The transition between normal and high pressure is quite easily seen when the septum does not move during inhalation, but moves from right to left with exhalation (if the patient is being mechanically ventilated). When the interatrial septum remains fixed left to right with ventilation, it is a sign of raised LAP (Kusumoto et al. 1993). When the atrium is empty, the movement of the interatrial septum is markedly increased in both directions through the cardiac cycle. The septum may appear concertinaed or buckled upon itself, and this reflects a low LAP. The best analogy is to think of the left atrium as a water-filled balloon. When the balloon is full of water and the pressure is high, it is circular in shape and if you cut a slice across the balloon, it would appear as a semicircle going outwards (i.e. the 'fixed curvature' seen with high LAP). If a small amount of water is let out, tapping the balloon on the edge with your hand would move the wall briefly inward before it sprang out again (i.e. the 'systolic reversal' seen with normal LAP). Finally, if the balloon is relatively empty, the walls will concertina or shrink down and appear to overlap, and a small tap of the hand will produce excessive motion (i.e. 'systolic buckling'). Figure 8.4 illustrates this method of estimating LAP for both TOE and TTE.

Royse et al. (2001) categorised these three states, and investigated how they change with the LAP. In a study performed in patients undergoing cardiopulmonary bypass, the shape and movement of the interatrial septum was observed while draining the blood out and then reinfusing it through the aortic cannula. They identified that the direction of change is proportional to the LAP; that is, as volume decreases the directional change is towards the lower LAP, and as volume increases, the LAP changes towards a higher state. The actual PCWP is less well defined by categorical measurements such as inter-atrial septal movement. As would be expected, there is a range of PCWP for each category, but in general terms, the trend in PCWP is in the same direction as the change in interatrial septal pattern.

The atrium is a 'window' to the LV. When there is LV diastolic dysfunction, the filling pressure in the left atrium must increase in order to fill the poorly compliant ventricle. As the pressure increases, the atrium will distend and appear balloon-shaped or 'unhappy' as

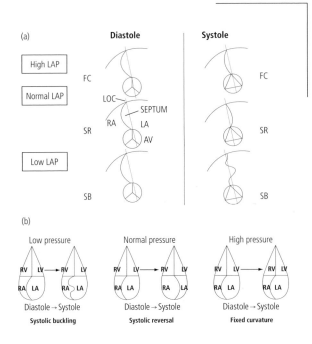

Figure 8.4 Estimating left atrial pressure by the interatrial septum method for (a) TOE and (b) TTE. SB: systolic buckling; SR: systolic reversal; FC: fixed curvature

described by Professor Terry Rafferty of Yale-New Haven Medical School. A large, tense and bulging left atrium looks 'unhappy', whereas a normal-sized chamber appears 'happy'. I strongly recommend that you, like Terry, become 'atrial watchers', because this very simple change has been shown to correlate with alterations in LAP.

Pulmonary vein Doppler: With a normal LAP, the proportion of flow in systole exceeds that in diastole, and as the LAP increases, the proportion changes so that the diastolic proportion predominates. What is generally poorly understood is that the relationship of the VTI of the pulmonary venous components rather than the peak

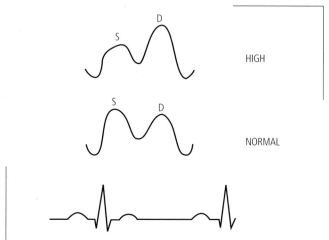

Figure 8.5 Estimating left atrial pressure from pulmonary vein flow

velocity is probably more accurate. A ratio of systolic to diastolic VTI <0.55 has been shown to correlate with PCWP >15 mmHg (Brunazzi et al. 1994; Kuecherer et al. 1990). An approximation of the ratio of systolic to diastolic peak velocities can be used, but has not been well validated against PCWP. It is quite easy to visually estimate the systolic and diastolic proportions of the pulmonary vein flow in order to identify a high LAP.

Step 4. Final Assessment
The key difference between echocardiography and invasive pressure monitoring for diagnosing the haemodynamic state is that echocardiography allows direct assessment of volume, systolic function and filling pressure. This combination of data enables an estimation of preload, ventricular function and, importantly, ventricular compliance. Only when compliance and volume are estimated together can diastolic heart failure be differentiated from the other haemodynamic states.

Table 8.1 is a guide to interpretation of the haemodynamic parameters observed in the 4-step basic assessment with regard to the seven basic states. The process is quite simple; for example, if preload

Table 8.1 Haemodynamic parameters

	Normal	Empty	Primary Diastolic Failure	Systolic Failure	Systolic & Diastolic Failure	Vasodilation	RV Failure
1. Volume	N	↓	N/↓	↑	↑	N	RV ↑
2. Systolic Function	N	N/↑	N	↓	↓	↑	RV ↓
3. Filling Pressure	N	↓	↑	N	↑	N	↑
4. Basic state	Normal	Empty	Primary Diastolic Failure	Systolic Failure	Systolic & Diastolic Failure	Vasodilation	RV Failure

is normal, function is normal and filling pressure is normal, then the first haemodynamic state has been defined; that is, 'normal'.

Normal haemodynamic state:	normal LVEDA, normal FAC, and normal LAP.
Empty (hypovolaemic):	reduced LVEDA, normal or increased FAC, and low LAP.
Primary diastolic failure:	reduced LVEDA (the ventricle will appear hypovolaemic), normal FAC, but high LAP. This haemodynamic state is very difficult to appreciate because it looks 'normal'. It is a conceptual leap to believe that a normal-looking ventricle constitutes heart failure. The key to identifying the state is to see a normal-looking ventricle operating at a high LAP.
Primary systolic failure:	increased LVEDA (dilated ventricle), reduced FAC, and normal LAP. Essentially, the compliance of the LV is normal or increased. It is important to differentiate dilated cardiomyopathy that is associated with normal LAP from that which is associated with increased LAP, because the haemodynamic performance may be quite different.
Systolic and diastolic failure:	increased LVEDA, reduced FAC, and increased LAP. These patients may represent the worst end of the heart failure spectrum, and may also have associated RV failure. The diastolic failure is evident by the raised LAP.

| Right ventricular failure: | dilated RV with reduced inward excursion, and elevated LAP. Although isolated RV failure can occur, it is frequently associated with LV failure. The RV will compress the LV, causing LV diastolic dysfunction (and the raised LAP). |

Figures 8.6 and 8.7 overleaf are an aide-mémoire of the 4-step basic haemodynamic assessment for TOE and TTE, respectively.

Value of haemodynamic diagnosis in patient management

The basic 4-step haemodynamic assessment enables the practitioner to determine the broad categories of haemodynamic abnormality, the treatments for which can be very different, even though the presenting signs and symptoms appear similar. The management of systolic failure appears straightforward, but that of diastolic failure is very different. For example, the use of an inodilator such as dobutamine or milrinone is standard therapy for patients with dilated cardiomyopathy and it appears logical that simultaneously increasing systolic function and facilitating ejection will improve global myocardial performance. However, the primary limitation in diastolic heart failure is reduced stroke volume because of reduced preload, rather than because of poor systolic function. Therefore, using an inodilator may reduce preload even further because of tachycardia (reduced filling time) and increased ejection fraction. The aim of this section is not to outline detailed therapeutic options, but rather to highlight that accurate diagnosis will lead to a logical choice of therapy. The exact choice of what type of infusion or what inotrope combination is best for each condition is largely a matter of experience and familiarity. I have outlined some broad categories of therapy for each of the seven haemodynamic states.

Normal	no need for therapy
Empty	infuse volume
Primary diastolic failure	maintain preload, control heart rate, treat concomitant vasodilation with a vasopressor, consider low-dose inotropes, but avoid high-dose inotropes if possible (see 'Systolic and diastolic failure' below)

Primary systolic failure	these patients are often quite stable under anaesthesia, but if global systolic performance is inadequate, they may benefit from inodilators
Systolic and diastolic failure	the key principle is to improve systolic performance at a reduced preload, which allows adequate cardiac output at a lower LAP. Therapy includes inodilators, increasing the heart rate (e.g. atrial pacing), decreasing preload by reducing volume infusion or by diuretics, and avoiding other therapies that may increase pressure around the heart (such as high levels of PEEP).
Vasodilation	vasoconstrictors
Right ventricular failure	very similar to the treatment for systolic and diastolic failure; inodilators such as dobutamine or milrinone improve RV systolic performance and also act as pulmonary vasodilators. Reducing RV pressure will reduce the compression of the LV, thereby improving its diastolic function. Consider pulmonary artery dilators, such as nitrates or nitric oxide, as part of the therapy regimen

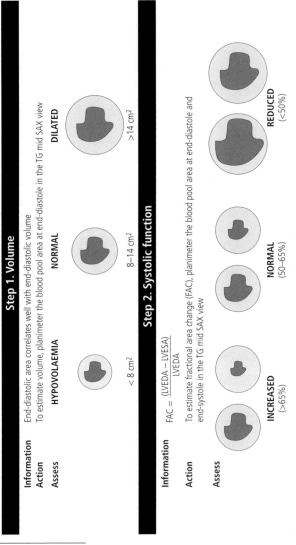

Step 1. Volume

Information End-diastolic area correlates well with end-diastolic volume

Action To estimate volume, planimeter the blood pool area at end-diastole in the TG mid SAX view

Assess

HYPOVOLAEMIA

< 8 cm²

NORMAL

8–14 cm²

DILATED

>14 cm²

Step 2. Systolic function

Information $FAC = \dfrac{(LVEDA - LVESA)}{LVEDA}$

Action To estimate fractional area change (FAC), planimeter the blood pool area at end-diastole and end-systole in the TG mid SAX view

Assess

INCREASED
(>65%)

NORMAL
(50–65%)

REDUCED
(<50%)

Figure 8.6 Basic 4-step haemodynamic assessment using TOE *continues*

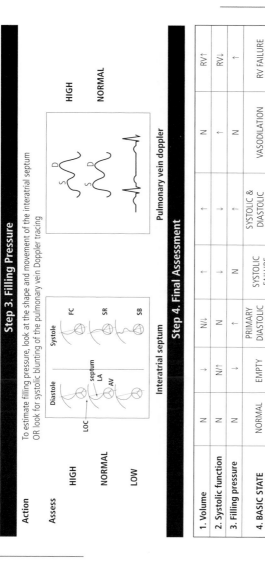

Step 3. Filling Pressure

Action

To estimate filling pressure, look at the shape and movement of the interatrial septum
OR look for systolic blunting of the pulmonary vein Doppler tracing

Assess

HIGH

NORMAL

LOW

Interatrial septum   Pulmonary vein doppler

Step 4. Final Assessment

1. Volume	N	→	N/↓	↑	N
2. Systolic function	N	N/↑	N	↓	↑
3. Filling pressure	N	→	↑	↑	N
4. BASIC STATE	NORMAL	EMPTY	PRIMARY DIASTOLIC FAILURE	SYSTOLIC FAILURE	SYSTOLIC & DIASTOLIC FAILURE	VASODILATION

RV↑
RV↓
↑
RV FAILURE

Figure 8.6 Basic 4-step haemodynamic assessment using TOE *continued*

Step 1. Volume

Information End-diastolic dimension correlates well with end-diastolic volume

Action In the PLAX view, place M-mode cursor across the LV base at chordae tendinae, perpendicular to the 2D interventricular septum and posterior wall, to obtain LVEDD at the onset of the QRS complex on ECG indexed to body surface area

Assess

HYPOVOLAEMIA	NORMAL	DILATED
<3 cm	3–5.6 cm	>5.6 cm

Step 2. Systolic function

Information $FS = \dfrac{LVEDD - LVESD}{LVEDD}$

Action In the PLAX view, place M-mode cursor through the base of the LV at the chordae tendinae, perpendicular to the 2D interventricular septum and posterior wall, to obtain LVEDD at the onset of the QRS wave and LVESD at the end of the T-wave on ECG

Assess

INCREASED	NORMAL	DECREASED
FS > 44%	FS 28–44%	FS < 28%

Figure 8.7 Basic 4-step haemodynamic assessment using TTE *continues*

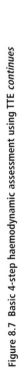

Step 3. Filling pressure

Action To estimate filling pressure, look at the shape and movement of interatrial septum in the apical 4-chamber view during the cardiac cycle

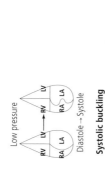

Low pressure

Diastole → Systole

Systolic buckling

Normal pressure

Diastole → Systole

Systolic reversal

High pressure

Diastole → Systole

Fixed curvature

Step 4. Final assessment

	NORMAL	EMPTY	PRIMARY DIASTOLIC FAILURE	SYSTOLIC FAILURE	SYSTOLIC & DIASTOLIC FAILURE	VASODILATION	RV FAILURE
1. Volume	N	→	N/↓	↑	↑	N	RV↑
2. Systolic function	N	N/↑	N	→	→	↑	RV↓
3. Filling pressure	N	→	↑	N	↑	N	↑
4. BASIC STATE	NORMAL	EMPTY	PRIMARY DIASTOLIC FAILURE	SYSTOLIC FAILURE	SYSTOLIC & DIASTOLIC FAILURE	VASODILATION	RV FAILURE

Figure 8.7 Basic 4-step haemodynamic assessment using TTE *continued*

Chapter 9
Problems with ventricles

Berthold Weitkamp

Learning objectives
1. Understand the common problems with ventricular function.
2. Understand how to use echocardiography to assess ventricular pathology.
3. Understand the use of echocardiography in ischaemic heart disease.
4. Understand the basic assessment and importance of diastolic function.
5. Understand the basic assessment of cardiomyopathies.
6. Understand the problems in diagnosing and interpreting cardiac masses.

Global ventricular function

Echocardiography is used for both qualitative and quantitative assessment of ventricular function. In clinical practice qualitative assessment is more common because quantitative measurements can be very time consuming and often do not add clinical value. An experienced operator will be able to assess the quality of contraction and the filling of the LV with minimal scanning time, which will assist in the management of fluid administration and inotropic treatment.

Assessment of ventricular function can be divided into global and regional assessment. Regional wall motion abnormalities (RWMAs) occur almost exclusively with ischaemic heart disease and will be discussed later in this chapter.

To assess global function, the TG mid SAX view (TOE) or the parasternal SAX view (TTE), angling laterally and inferiorly, sweeping from the basal to apical sections of the LV, should be obtained. These views are reproducible and suitable for repeated measurements of filling. The distribution of the three major coronary arteries can be seen. From the TG mid SAX (TOE) or parasternal SAX papillary muscle level (TTE), an assessment of the size of the LV can then be made; that is, small, normal or dilated. Inward movement and thickening of the ventricular walls can be observed and systolic function can be estimated. It is useful to imagine the centre point of the LV cavity and determine whether all the walls move and thicken to the same degree. Three grades of wall motion have been described, based on the degree of radial shortening or the ejection fraction (EF) estimate. Although the EF is affected by alterations in loading condition, in clinical practice it is a fairly reliable indicator of global systolic function: EF >65% is considered normal, 50–65% low normal, 40–50% mildly reduced, 30–40% moderately reduced, <30% severely reduced global systolic function. The fractional area change (FAC) gives similar values, but fractional shortening (FS) is proportionally less with FS >30% considered normal and 25% as reduced.

Assessment of left ventricular function

Fractional area change: When using TOE, the FAC is a reliable and rapidly obtained index of global systolic function. In the TG mid SAX view, the freeze and scroll functions are used to find the largest (end-diastolic) frame and the smallest (end-systolic) frame. The endocardial surfaces can then be traced to measure the end-diastolic area (EDA) and end-systolic area (ESA):

$$FAC = \frac{EDA - ESA}{EDA} \times 100$$

Normal values are EDA <14 cm^2, ESA <6 cm^2, and FAC 60%. Other quantitative measurements include FS, EF, SV and CO and circumferential fibre shortening.

When using TTE, all measurements are performed in the PLAX view and FS is calculated (see Chapter 8).

Assessing right ventricular function

The ventricles have a close anatomical and functional relationship. The RV and LV dimensions can be compared in the MO 4-chamber view (TOE), or the apical 4-chamber or subcostal 4-chamber view (TTE).

Normally, the RV is approximately two-thirds of the size of the LV; with mild dilatation it is still smaller than the LV, but when dilated it is the same size and when severely dilated the RV is larger than the LV.

Extension of the RV towards the apex of the heart can also be used as a marker for dilatation: normally the RV extends two-thirds towards the apex, a dilated RV reaches the apex, and a severely dilated RV extends beyond the apex.

Causes of RV dilatation include:

- Pressure overload—pulmonary hypertension or pulmonary stenosis
- Volume overload—either valvular regurgitation or left-to-right shunt
- RV failure—ischaemic heart disease or as a consequence of pressure or volume overload.

Because of its anatomical position and non-uniform shape, the function of the RV is much harder to assess than that of the LV. No reliable quantitative method has been described, but a qualitative assessment can be made. Observing the contraction of the free wall will give most of the information needed. Subtle dysfunction may be difficult to determine, but signs of severe RV failure are:

- Akinesis of the free wall
- Rounded shape
- Interventricular septum curved to the left.

Ischaemic heart disease

Both TTE and TOE are helpful in diagnosing suspected ischaemic heart disease and further defining the stage of the disease process. They have also become a common tool in clinical decision-making.

The signs of myocardial ischaemia and infarction that can be diagnosed by echocardiography include:

- Regional wall motion abnormality
- Dilated ischaemic cardiomyopathy
- Mitral regurgitation (often dynamic in severity)

- Papillary muscle rupture or dysfunction
- Ventricular septal rupture
- Ventricular aneurysm
- Ventricular pseudoaneurysm
- Ventricular free wall rupture.

Ischaemic cardiomyopathy is characterised by severe global systolic and diastolic dysfunction. The LV is dilated and RWMAs may be present. Often the myocardium appears thin and poorly contracting. Intramural thrombi should be excluded (see later section).

Mitral regurgitation (MR) may be a consequence of acute LV 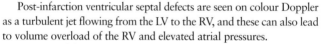 dysfunction caused by myocardial ischaemia. It is also a good marker for the severity of LV dysfunction after cardiopulmonary bypass. The areas of the LV that are most commonly involved are the inferior and posterior walls. Severe MR can be also caused by a papillary muscle rupture, in which case flail mitral segments are usually seen passing into the LA during systole, resulting in severe haemodynamic instability. In less severe cases the papillary muscle may not have completely ruptured, but LV dysfunction occurs because of the transient ischaemia.

Post-infarction ventricular septal defects are seen on colour Doppler as a turbulent jet flowing from the LV to the RV, and these can also lead to volume overload of the RV and elevated atrial pressures.

Rupture of the ventricular free wall can cause either sudden death from acute cardiac tamponade or development of a pseudoaneurysm. The pseudoaneurysm is only lined with pericardium and requires urgent surgical repair. Look for a narrow neck (less than half the size of the aneurysm) and thrombus in the cavity should be excluded.

In contrast, a true post-infarction ventricular aneurysm is lined with thin, non-contractile myocardium. It is mainly scar tissue and there is usually no danger of rupture. However, depending on its size, acute LV dysfunction can occur. Characteristics of an aneurysm include a wide neck (more than half the size of the aneurysm), a smooth transition from contractile myocardium to scar tissue, and spontaneous echo contrast ('smoke'). There may be a thrombus.

Cardiomyopathies

The term 'cardiomyopathy' describes a group of primary myocardial diseases that are classified by their dominant pathophysiology: dilated

cardiomyopathy, restrictive cardiomyopathy, and hypertrophic
cardiomyopathy.

Dilated cardiomyopathy

The main echocardiographic finding is systolic cardiac failure. The LV
is dilated with reduced EF. The atria may be enlarged and SEC may
be seen. Thrombi in the left atrial appendage (LAA) should be
excluded. Ventricular mural thrombi are also common. MR and TR
may occur because of annular dilatation. The prognosis largely
depends on the degree of dilatation rather than the degree of systolic
dysfunction.

Restrictive cardiomyopathy

In contrast to dilated cardiomyopathy, the main echocardiographic
finding is diastolic cardiac failure (Figure 9.1). Systolic function and
LV size are usually preserved until late in the disease process. Both
atria may dilate, and MR and TR may occur. Hypertrophy of the LV
will also occur in the later stages of the disease.

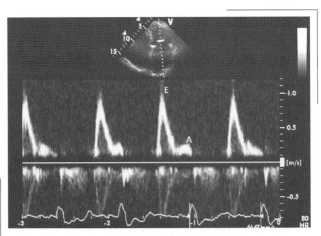

Figure 9.1 Mitral inflow PW Doppler showing a restrictive filling profile

Hypertrophic cardiomyopathy

The main characteristic is hypertrophy of the LV wall (most commonly, the septum). Often the upper (basal) portion of the septum is involved, causing narrowing of the LVOT, which in 25% of patients results in dynamic outflow obstruction and the disease is then called hypertrophic obstructive cardiomyopathy or idiopathic hypertrophic subaortic stenosis.

Echocardiographic findings include normal or hyperdynamic LV systolic function, septal hypertrophy, diastolic dysfunction with high filling pressures, systolic anterior motion (SAM) of the MV with resultant eccentric MR, and a typical dagger-shaped (late systolic peak) Doppler profile of the obstructive flow (Figure 9.2). This characteristic appearance aids in differentiating the waveform from coexisting MR or an aortic stenotic jet.

The SAM of the MV is thought to be caused by the Venturi effect of high-speed blood flow through the LVOT. The anterior mitral valve leaflet is 'pulled' anteriorly, resulting in LVOT outflow obstruction, which may also lead to posteriorly directed MR. The treatment for SAM consists of rate and contractility control (i.e. beta-blockade), and increased preload and afterload.

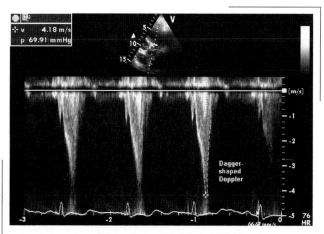

Figure 9.2 Typical dagger-shaped CW Doppler profile of HCM

The echocardiography examination will guide the treatment and fluid management of patients with HCM. First, the location and extent of septal thickening should be assessed and measured. Second, the degree of SAM and MR needs to be evaluated. Third, the pressure gradient across the LVOT should be assessed in either the deep TG LAX or TG LAX views for TOE, or apical 5-chamber view for TTE using CW Doppler. Occasionally, a patient may display typical HOCM characteristics on echocardiography without a significant LVOT gradient. The gradient may be worsened by employing the Valsalva manoeuvre.

Surgical treatment of HOCM includes septal myomectomy and it is important to exclude a ventricular septal defect post procedure.

Regional wall motion abnormalities

RWMAs can be defined as regions of the LV that are performing at different grades of systolic function. In most cases this will be caused by ischaemic heart disease, but other causes include myocardial infarction, myocardial stunning, intercoronary air and imperfect coronary grafts. There is increasing evidence that echocardiography is a more sensitive monitor for cardiac ischaemia than the surface 5-lead ECG and will detect more ischaemic events up to several minutes earlier than ECG. TOE has therefore become the method of choice for continuous intraoperative ischaemia monitoring in cardiac and other high-risk surgery.

Analysis of RWMA

The 17-segment model of the LV is used to identify and locate RWMAs (see Chapter 4). It is important to complete the full examination and interrogate the LV with all available views.

The grading of severity of dysfunction is summarised in Table 9.1. It is important to look for myocardial thickening rather than endocardial movement alone.

A change in the degree of dysfunction can be difficult to diagnose. Worsening of segmental wall motion by at least two grades is required to diagnose acute ischaemia. Smaller changes in regional function cannot be reliably interpreted.

After an initial complete examination, the TG mid SAX view is used for continuous monitoring of myocardial ischaemia. As

Table 9.1 Grade of regional wall motion abnormality

Class	Wall thickening	Change in radius
1. Normal	Marked	>30% decrease
2. Mild hypokinesis	Moderate	10–30% decrease
3. Severe hypokinesis	Minimal	0–10% decrease
4. Akinesis	None	None
5. Dyskinesis	Thinning	Outward movement of segment

mentioned, this transverse plane view through the mid portion of both papillary muscles includes myocardium supplied by all three coronary arteries and any new wall motion abnormalities can be evaluated. Note that some wall motion abnormalities (20%) can only be picked up in the LAX views of the LV. Because continuous multiplane analysis is not yet available, the TG mid SAX view remains the best choice.

Interpretation of RWMA

The cause of RWMAs is predominantly myocardial ischaemia, although other causes have been described. Myocardial stunning is a condition occurring after ischaemia, infarction or cardiopulmonary bypass. Stunned myocardium appears akinetic, but responds to inotropes, whereas the function of infarcted tissue will not improve.

Myocardial infarction will commonly produce a segment of akinesis or dyskinesis. Given sufficient time after infarction the myocardium may 'remodel' and present as a thin and dilated area of the wall, which may also develop into an aneurysm.

Intracoronary air may also cause transient RWMAs after open heart surgery. The inferior wall is mainly affected because the right coronary artery is the most anterior of the coronary arteries.

Other causes of RWMAS include hypovolaemia, epicardial pacing, left bundle branch block, severe MR and imperfect coronary bypass grafts.

Assessing diastolic function

In recent years the clinical importance of diastolic dysfunction has been recognised. Many patients present to the cardiologist in heart failure, but with normal or near normal systolic function. Diastolic heart failure is also commonly found in cardiac surgery patients. Diastolic dysfunction can lead to significant haemodynamic disturbances, particularly in the post-bypass period.

Diastolic dysfunction is defined as a condition in which the heart (mainly the LV) cannot fill adequately during diastole. The myocardium is too 'stiff' and cannot relax, leading to increased filling pressures. Early myocardial relaxation is an active process requiring energy and is dependent on adequate blood supply. Therefore, ischaemic heart disease is a common cause. Impaired ventricular filling may also result from other conditions such as pericardial tamponade, constrictive pericarditis, LV hypertrophy or amyloidosis.

Echocardiography has become an important tool in the assessment of diastolic function. In the OR, diastolic function should be assessed pre and post cardiopulmonary bypass, because early inotropic intervention in severe diastolic dysfunction with near normal systolic function can often prevent haemodynamic problems and will reduce complications when 'weaning' from bypass.

The common echocardiographic measurements used to assess diastolic function are semi-quantitative and their accuracy is often dependent on heart rhythm and filling state. A more simplistic assessment of diastolic function is explained in Chapter 8. At least two of the three different methods of imaging described next are needed in order to form a meaningful conclusion.

Mitral inflow pattern

In the MO 4-chamber (TOE) or apical 4-chamber (TTE) view, the cursor is positioned just distal to the MV at the level of the leaflet tips and PW Doppler is used. In patients with a heart rate of less than 80 beats/min and normal sinus rhythm, there will be two characteristic waves: the E wave and the A wave. The E wave represents early ventricular filling after the MV opens and the A wave represents filling of the LV during atrial contraction.

The E and A wave peak velocities, deceleration time (DT) of the E wave and the duration of the A wave are measured (Figure 9.3). The DT is derived from the slope of the descent of the E wave. This

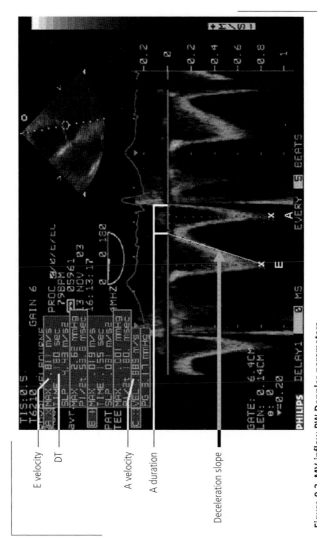

Figure 9.3 MV inflow PW Doppler parameters

important measurement of the deceleration of flow across the MV is inversely related to LV compliance. A 'stiff' ventricle will have a short DT, whereas a slowly relaxing ventricle with mild stiffness will have a prolonged DT.

There are four distinct patterns of MV inflow (Figure 9.4):

- Normal inflow (E > A, DT 150–220 ms, normal LAP)
- Abnormal relaxation (E < A, DT >220 ms, normal LAP)
- Pseudonormal (E > A, DT 150–220 ms, high LAP)
- Restrictive filling (E >> A, DT <150 ms, high LAP).

The pathological filling patterns can also be regarded as grades of severity, with abnormal relaxation being the mildest form of dysfunction and restrictive filling being the most severe, although restrictive filling is seen more commonly with dilated cardiomyopathy than with diastolic heart failure (normal EF). The differentiation between the grades is not always clearly defined. In patients over 65 years of age equalisation of the E and A wave velocities occurs, but as the LV gets 'stiffer', the LAP will rise and re-establish the pressure gradient between the LA and LV. The mitral inflow pattern will look normal again because the E wave has become prominent. To distinguish between 'normal' and 'pseudonormal' two other parameters are taken into account: LAP and pulmonary venous inflow PW Doppler.

Left atrial pressure: The movement and shape of the interatrial septum can be used to estimate LAP. With normal LAP, the septum is curved left or right except during mid systole when it reverses, causing a 'flip flop' motion with each cardiac cycle. As LAP increases, the curve remains fixed towards the right throughout the cardiac cycle. This method cannot be used in patients with severe TR or MR because the bowing of the septum will be related to this pathology and not to atrial filling.

Pulmonary venous inflow pattern

Pulsed wave Doppler of the pulmonary venous inflow is best obtained in either the MO 2- or 4-chamber view (TOE) or apical 4-chamber view (TTE). The left upper pulmonary vein is usually well positioned for interrogation and is found by leftward rotation from either of the the views for TOE. The right upper pulmonary vein is usually interrogated using TTE. To confirm the correct position of the cursor, CFD can be used.

normal

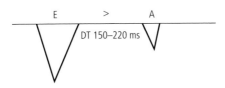

abnormal relaxation pattern

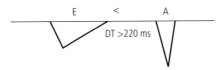

pseudonormal pattern

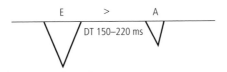

restrictive pattern

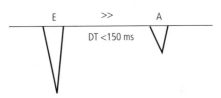

Figure 9.4 Summary of MV filling patterns

Pulse wave Doppler of the inflow will produce three distinct waves:

- Systolic (S) wave (towards the apex)—represents flow into the LA during atrial relaxation and downward movement of the MV in systole
- Diastolic (D) wave—represents the passive inflow after the opening of the MV
- Atrial reversal (Ar)—represents reversal of flow during atrial systole.

The S wave is greater than the D wave, and the peak Ar velocity is less than 0.35 m/s. In general, it can be postulated that with increasing LAP and worsening of diastolic function the S wave will become blunted, the D wave will become more prominent and the Ar velocity will increase. A high LAP helps to differentiate between normal (Figure 9.5) and pseudonormal flow (Figure 9.6).

Blunting of the S wave also occurs from other causes of high LAP, including poor systolic function, MR and atrial fibrillation.

A useful 'rule of thumb' for interpreting diastolic function is that diastolic dysfunction is unlikely to be severe if the LAP is normal, and is likely to be clinically important if the LAP is high.

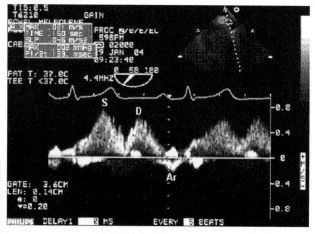

Figure 9.5 Normal PV Doppler profile

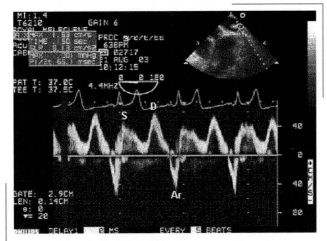

Figure 9.6 Abnormal PV Doppler profile. The D wave is greater than the S wave and atrial reversal velocity is >35 cm/s

Tissue Doppler imaging

TDI is a relatively new method of assessing diastolic function. Its main value is that the measurement is relatively pre-load and heart-rate independent. TDI measures the myocardial wall motion velocity. Normal myocardial wall motion velocity is 10 cm/s, but has a much higher amplitude than blood flow. Therefore, the TDI presets adjust the scale, wall filter and gain settings in order to detect velocities less than 20 cm/s.

TDI is best used in the MO 2- or 4-chamber views (TOE) or the apical 4-chamber view (TTE). The view chosen is one that gives best parallel alignment with the Doppler signal. By placing the cursor just below the MV over the myocardium of the ventricular free wall, a spectral PW signal of myocardial velocity can be displayed. A typical display consists of the early diastolic E wave (E') and a late diastolic A wave (A'). It has been established that E' velocities of greater than 8 cm/s are associated with normal diastolic function (Figure 9.7) and values less than that are indicative of diastolic dysfunction (Figure 9.8), but it can not be predicted whether the dysfunction is abnormal relaxation, pseudonormal or restrictive.

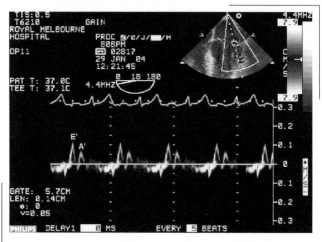

Figure 9.7 Normal TDI (TOE). The early diastolic E wave (E') is approximately 11 cm/s

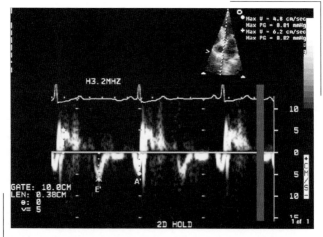

Figure 9.8 Abnormal TDI (TTE). The early diastolic E wave (E') is approximately 6 cm/s (Ap4ch view shows an inverted wave profile compared with Figure 9.7)

Cardiac masses and locating a potential cardiac source of embolus

The use of TOE for identifying intracardiac masses and locating possible sources of emboli is well established in clinical practice. A cardiac mass can be defined as an abnormal structure within or immediately adjacent to the heart, such as a tumour, thrombus, vegetations or a foreign body. It is sometimes difficult to identify a cardiac mass and in some cases identification is extremely operator-dependent. Ultrasound artifacts and several normal structures may be mistaken for a cardiac mass (see Chapter 3).

The following rules should be followed to identify a mass:
- The mass should be examined throughout the cardiac cycle.
- More than one view should be used.
- The findings need to be interpreted in view of the patient's clinical picture (i.e. endocarditis, stroke etc.)

Once a cardiac mass has been identified it has to be determined whether it is most likely to be a tumour, vegetation or thrombus.

Thrombus

A thrombus can form in regions of low velocity blood flow or blood stasis. This can occur in any chamber of the heart but right heart thrombi are very rare.

Left ventricle: Severe LV dysfunction, RWMAs, ventricular aneurysms or pseudoaneurysms are all associated with the formation of thrombi. TTE is usually superior in detecting thrombi in the LV, especially in the apex (Figure 9.9).

Left atrium: Left atrial thrombi are associated with atrial enlargement, MV stenosis and atrial fibrillation. In cases of poor LV function a thrombus can develop in the atrium even when sinus rhythm is preserved. The LAA is the most likely site for a thrombus. A thrombus should always be excluded when SEC is present. Because of the proximity of the atrium to the probe TOE has a much greater sensitivity and negative predictive value for LA thrombi than LV thrombi. The LAA is usually well seen in the MO 2-chamber view (Figure 9.10). The angle it is best seen at varies between $0°$ and $90°$. It is common practice to exclude a LA thrombus before cardioverting a patient with chronic atrial fibrillation.

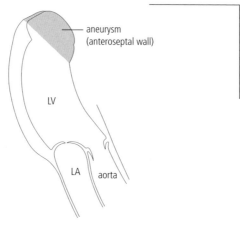

Figure 9.9 Apical aneurysm (TTE, apical LAX)

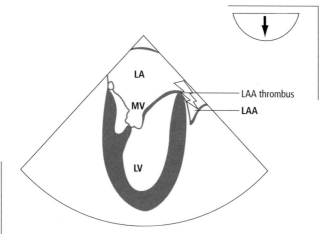

Figure 9.10 Thrombus in LAA (TOE, MO 2-chamber)

Vegetations

Vegetations are a frequent consequence of endocarditis and TOE is the investigation of choice for this condition. The TOE findings will often determine whether surgery is indicated.

Vegetations are irregular in shape, usually globular and often pedunculated. The risk of embolisation increases with size. Vegetations greater than 1 cm have a 50% risk of shearing off and causing embolism.

Vegetations usually occur on the mitral and aortic valves and are usually attached to the upstream side of the valve. Severe regurgitation is a frequent finding. Right-sided vegetations occur in patients with intravenous drug abuse and may require replacement of the TV because of the severe regurgitation.

It is important to identify paravalvular abscesses, which may also present as a cardiac mass.

Cardiac tumours

Compared with lung or brain tumours, cardiac tumours are rare. Secondary tumours are 20-fold more common than primary cardiac tumours.

Primary cardiac tumours: The most common primary cardiac tumour is the benign myxoma, comprising approximately 27% of all adult primary cardiac tumours, of which 75% occur in the left atrium, 18% in the right atrium and 4% in each of the ventricles.

Their appearance can vary from circumscribed to irregular. Typically, a LA myxoma presents as a mobile echogenic mass (Figure 9.12a, b) that may partially pass through the MV in diastole, obstructing LV filling. Myxomas can be surprisingly large and can occupy almost all of the atrium.

Papillary fibroelastoma comprises approximately 13% of all primary cardiac tumours (Figure 9.13). It is much smaller than a myxoma and is usually attached to the downstream side of the mitral or aortic valve. It is usually pedunculated and can mimic a vegetation, and embolisation can occur.

Other primary cardiac tumours include lipoma, rhabdomyoma (mainly in children), fibroma and sarcomas.

Secondary cardiac tumours: Tumours can affect the heart either by direct invasion (i.e. lung and breast), or lymphatic or metastatic spread. Most common are lung metastases followed by lymphoma, breast, leukaemia, GI tract, melanoma and liver tumours. Melanomas have the highest rate of pericardial spread, but lung tumours are far more frequent. The tumours can invade the myocardium (lymphoma

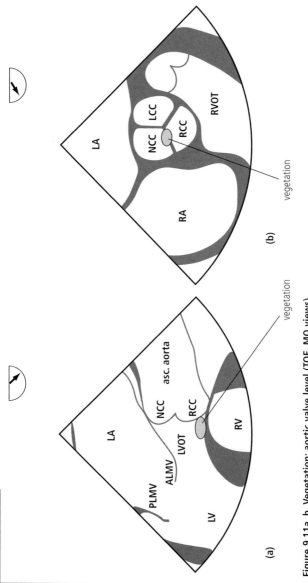

Figure 9.11a, b Vegetation: aortic valve level (TOE, MO views)

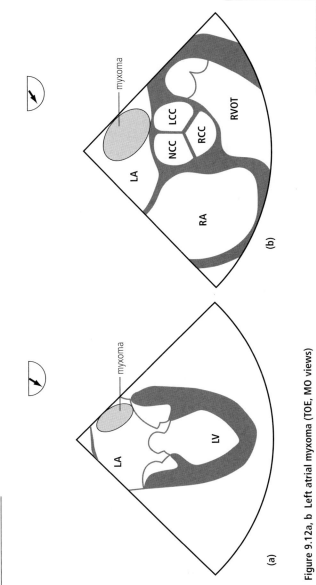

Figure 9.12a, b Left atrial myxoma (TOE, MO views)

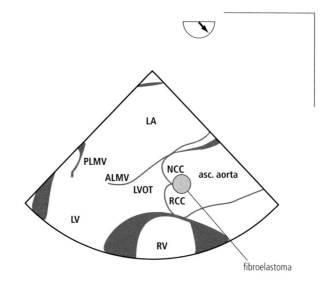

Figure 9.13 Aortic valve fibroelastoma (TOE, MO aortic valve LAX)

and melanoma), grow within any chamber, and cause cardiovascular disturbance. The pericardium is frequently involved and a malignant pericardial effusion carries a high mortality. The endocardium is rarely involved. Renal cell carcinoma can invade the right atrium, and it can be followed down the IVC to the kidneys via the subcostal approach during TTE.

Chapter 10
Problems with valves

Peter Dawson

Learning objectives
1. Understand common valve problems.
2. Understand the use of echocardiography in the assessment of valve disease.
3. Understand the assessment of prosthetic valves.
4. Understand the role of echocardiography in suspected endocarditis.

Aortic valve

Aortic stenosis

Aortic stenosis (AS) arises from degenerative, congenital, rheumatic, and endocarditic causes. In 70–80% of cases there is also aortic regurgitation (AR).

Degenerative calcific AS is most common in patients over the age of 70 years, with 1–2% of these cases having concomitant subaortic stenosis secondary to muscular obstruction. There is leaflet thickening, and calcification arising from the leaflet base. Stiffening of the valve creates a funnel-shaped opening.

Congenital causes of AS include a bicuspid valve and, rarely, unicommissural unicuspid and acommissural unicuspid valves. Unicuspid valves are usually detected as AS in childhood and exhibit leaflet doming (MO AV LAX view (TOE), PLAX (TTE)).

Bicuspid valves are the commonest cause of AS in patients under 70 years of age, occurring in 1–2% of the population, and in males they are usually associated with aortic coarctation, ventricular septal defects, atrial septal defects and pulmonic stenosis. Half the cases have an anteroposterior orientation with fusion of the vestigial left and right cusps, with the coronaries arising from this larger, anterior leaflet. In the lateromedial variety, coronaries arise from both the left and the larger right cusp. Bicuspid valves calcify and often have a prominent raphe in the larger leaflet, which makes it difficult to distinguish them from calcified trileaflet valves. There may be post-stenotic dilatation of the ascending aorta. The echocardiographer must identify the coronary origin and associated pathology.

Rheumatic fever results in fibrosis, calcification and fusion of the edges of the valve leaflets, which results in doming of the leaflets during systole. Other valves may be affected, particularly the MV.

Causes of subaortic stenosis, such as a subaortic membrane, hypertrophic obstructive cardiomyopathy and SAM, must be excluded.

In response to AS, the LV develops concentric hypertrophy (LVH) to minimise wall tension. As the disease progresses, the LV dilates, mitral regurgitation (MR) may develop, and finally, pulmonary hypertension and right heart failure occurs. In 50% of patients there is associated coronary artery disease. Combined AV replacement with coronary artery grafting has become a common operation in many cardiac units.

Echocardiographic assessment of aortic stenosis

Qualitative: Valve leaflets can be assessed in the MO AV SAX and MO AV LAX views (TOE), and the PLAX and PSAX views (TTE). The deep TG TOE views are useful if calcification obscures the subvalvular structures. When using CFD, aliasing is seen in the ascending aorta because of the high velocity jet and turbulence. The velocity can be measured by CW Doppler. An increased LV wall thickness indicates LVH, whereas increased LV diameter, area or volume indicates LV dilatation. There may be diastolic dysfunction consequent to the development of LVH.

Quantitative: Severity can be measured by gradient, jet velocity or aortic valve area (Table 10.1). Severe or moderate AS accompanied by moderate to severe AR in symptomatic patients requires valve replacement. Peak velocity is used to follow the progression of AS because the observer variability is 0.1%. Observer error using AVA is >0.15 cm^2, mainly because of error in the measurement of the LVOT

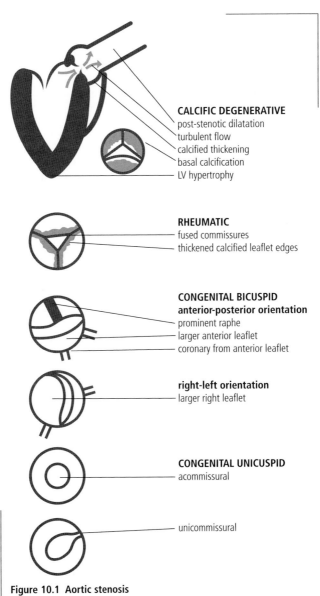

CALCIFIC DEGENERATIVE
post-stenotic dilatation
turbulent flow
calcified thickening
basal calcification
LV hypertrophy

RHEUMATIC
fused commissures
thickened calcified leaflet edges

CONGENITAL BICUSPID
anterior–posterior orientation
prominent raphe
larger anterior leaflet
coronary from anterior leaflet

right–left orientation
larger right leaflet

CONGENITAL UNICUSPID
acommissural

unicommissural

Figure 10.1 Aortic stenosis

Table 10.1 Quantification of aortic stenosis

Grade	Area (cm²)	Area/BSA (cm²/m²)	Mean gradient (mmHg)
Normal	3–5		
Mild	1.0–1.5	>0.8	<20
Moderate	0.8–1.0	0.5–0.8	21–49
Severe	<0.8	<0.5	>50

diameter (an error that is squared). AS typically worsens 0.1 cm² per year (0–0.5 cm²).

Aortic regurgitation

Aortic regurgitation may be caused by abnormalities of the aortic valve leaflets, aortic root, or a combined process affecting both root and valve leaflets.

Leaflet abnormality is most common with bicuspid valves, rheumatic fever, endocarditis, trauma or degenerative calcific aortic valve disease associated with ageing. The cusps should be interrogated for perforation, prolapse, retraction, or loss of basal support.

Aortic root pathology causes dilatation of the aortic commissures or annulus, and failure of leaflet coaptation. Causes include ascending aortic aneurysm, aortic dissection, mycotic aneurysm, annuloaortic ectasia, cystic medial necrosis and, rarely, osteogenesis imperfecta or Behcet syndrome.

Combined leaflet and aortic root disease includes Marfan's syndrome, chronic hypertension and, rarely, syphilis.

Echocardiographic assessment of aortic regurgitation

Echocardiographic evaluation of AR involves an assessment of the mechanism and then quantification (Table 10.2). An increased dimension of the aortic root, abnormal leaflet morphology and poor coaptation may identify the diagnosis. Severe AR is associated with holodiastolic flow reversal in the descending aorta (Figure 10.3), a dense CW Doppler signal in the regurgitant jet, a restrictive mitral flow pattern if acute (decreased DT of the E wave), and in chronic AR the LV diastolic diameter is greater than 7.5 cm. Mild AR may have early diastolic flow reversal in the descending aorta, a faint CW signal and, in chronic AR, the LV diastolic diameter is greater than 6.0 cm.

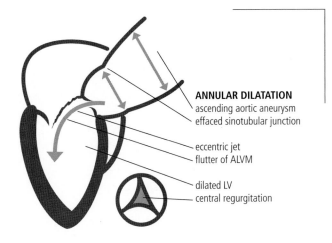

ANNULAR DILATATION
ascending aortic aneurysm
effaced sinotubular junction

eccentric jet
flutter of ALVM

dilated LV
central regurgitation

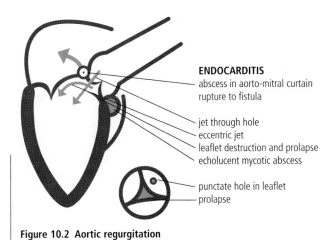

ENDOCARDITIS
abscess in aorto-mitral curtain
rupture to fistula

jet through hole
eccentric jet
leaflet destruction and prolapse
echolucent mycotic abscess

punctate hole in leaflet
prolapse

Figure 10.2 Aortic regurgitation

(a)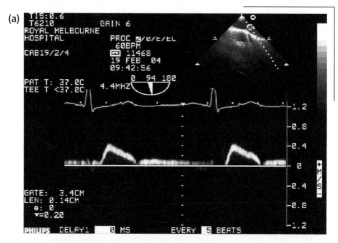

(b)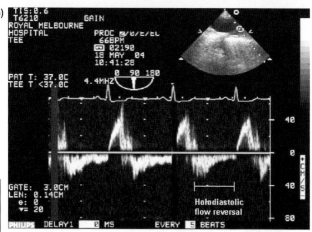

Holodiastolic
flow reversal

Figure 10.3 Descending aorta showing (a) normal flow and (b)
holodiastolic flow reversal consistent with severe AR

Table 10.2 Quantification of aortic regurgitation

Grade	AR jet area/ LVOT area (%)	Regurgitant fraction (%)	Jet height/ LVOT height (%)	Pressure half-time (ms)
Mild	<30	<30	<30	>400
Moderate	30–60	30–55	30–60	250–400
Severe	>60	>55	>60	<250

Mitral valve

Mitral stenosis

Stenosis of the MV may be caused by rheumatic fever, degenerative calcification, left atrial myxoma or congenital causes (Figure 10.4).

Rheumatic valves show commissural fusion, which restricts the edges of the leaflets during diastole, resulting in bowing or doming of the body of the leaflets into the LV ('hockey stick' appearance). The edges are thickened, fibrotic and may show islets of calcification. Chordae are shortened, thickened, fibrotic and calcified, and may rupture.

Mitral annular calcification is a degenerative age-related process (>60 years). Calcification of the posterior annulus may progress to the anterior annulus and extend from the base of the valve leaflets as ridges that restrict valve movement. Leaflet edges are normal without commissural fusion and the annulus is echodense with acoustic shadowing beyond.

Atrial myxoma may obstruct the mitral orifice and mimic MS.

Echocardiographic assessment of mitral stenosis

The LA is enlarged and the LV appears under-filled. Using CFD reveals a high-velocity jet into the LV with LA flow convergence. Elevated LAP results in fixed bowing of the interatrial septum to the right, pulmonary venous hypertension extending to pulmonary artery hypertension, and dilation of the RA and RV. The pulmonary hypertension may become irreversible. TR may occur secondary to tricuspid annular dilatation, and MR may also be present. Low flow in the LA appears as a swirling echo-dense pattern in the LA chamber ('smoke'), and subsequently a laminated thrombus or LAA thrombus may develop (see Chapter 9).

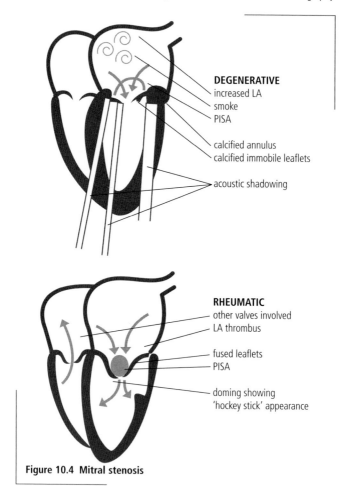

DEGENERATIVE
increased LA
smoke
PISA

calcified annulus
calcified immobile leaflets

acoustic shadowing

RHEUMATIC
other valves involved
LA thrombus

fused leaflets
PISA

doming showing
'hockey stick' appearance

Figure 10.4 Mitral stenosis

The outcome of commissurotomy is most favourable where there is fusion without fibrosis or calcification, no MR, and no LA thrombus.

Quantification of MS can be made by gradient or area (see Chapter 7 and Table 10.3). Low flow across the valve because of the severity of the MS may result in lower than expected gradients, and

Table 10.3 Quantification of mitral stenosis

Grade	Mean gradient (mmHg)	Pressure half-time (ms) MVA = 220/PHT	MVA (cm²) Continuity equation or PISA
Normal	<6	30–60	4–6
Mild	6	100–150	1.5–2
Moderate	6–12	150–200	1.0–1.5
Severe	>12	>200	<1.0

exercise or a hyperdynamic state may increase the gradient. The area of the MV (MVA) is independent of transmitral flow. The presence of atrial fibrillation requires averaging of 6–9 cardiac cycles to improve accuracy.

Planimetry can be used to directly measure MVA by tracing the edges of the MV leaflets, but the funnel shape of the valve makes it difficult to define the leaflet edge.

Mitral regurgitation
The function of the MV can be directly affected by alteration to any one of its components (i.e. anterior and posterior leaflets, annulus, chordae) and indirectly by disease of its attachments (i.e. LV, LA or papillary muscles). The aetiology of MR can often be identified with echocardiography (e.g. myxomatous and rheumatic valves), but many features overlap the different aetiologies, allowing only a description of the mechanism.

Carpentier grouped MV pathology as:
- Normal leaflets—annular dilatation caused by LA or LV dilatation, secondary to cardiomyopathy or ischaemic heart disease.
- Abnormal leaflets with prolapse—chordal elongation, ruptured chords, ruptured papillary muscle or myxomatous degeneration of leaflets.
- Abnormal leaflets with restriction—rheumatic valve, chordal shortening because of ischaemia, globular-shaped LV from remodelling or cardiomyopathy leading to lateral displacement of the papillary muscles.

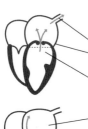

PROLAPSE
pulmonary flow reversal
bileaflet prolapse above annular line
thick leaflet, rolled edges is myxomatous
central regurgitant jet
dilated annulus

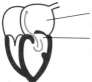

single leaflet prolapse
may have thickened myxomatous leaflet
eccentric jet entrains blood on one side of its tail
PISA hemisphere

FLAIL
ruptured chordae
flail leaflet
eccentric jet away from abnormal leaflet
may be degenerative with calcification of annulus
acoustic shadow

DILATED ANNULUS
enlarged atrium
smoke
LAA thrombus
dilated annulus
central regurgitant jet with failed central coaptation
dilated LV with reduced systolic function
apically displaced PAP muscles

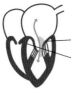

RESTRICTED—RHEUMATIC
dilated annulus
retracted thickened leaflets
thick short chords
doming, possible MS and other valves

FLAIL—ACUTE ISCHAEMIC
pulmonary flow reversal and APO
ruptured PAP muscle
flail leaflet
normal chamber size
dyskinetic LV
thrombus

Figure 10.5 Mitral regurgitation

Echocardiographic assessment of mitral regurgitation

The mechanism and severity of MR determines the choice of surgical repair or replacement.

Valve leaflets: Myxomatous leaflets are thickened and redundant, flopping into the atrium during systole. The leaflet edges roll, increasing the echocardiographic appearance of thickening. Rheumatic leaflets show commissural thickening. Endocarditis is characterised by leaflets with punctate holes, and granulomas on the LA side. Long, redundant anterior leaflets are associated with Marfan's syndrome. Degenerative MR has similar features to degenerative MS.

Annulus, left atrium and left ventricle: Normally, the mitral valve bows towards the LA and becomes smaller during systole. Annular calcification (in degenerative MR) prevents this. Calcification is frequently seen in the posterior annulus as an arc, which in severe cases extends anteriorly onto the valve leaflets and into the LV, interfering with chordal attachments. Echocardiographic features include acoustic shadowing extending beyond bright echodense structures that persist even after reducing the gain. Calcification is seen in renal failure, hypertension, and degeneration associated with ageing.

Endocarditis may result in abscess formation, destruction of the fibroskeleton or communication between chambers around the fibroskeleton, producing paravalvular MR.

Dilatation of the LA or LV may cause a central jet of MR because of the annular dilatation and failure of coaptation of the leaflets.

Leaflet motion and coaptation: Normally, coaptation of valve leaflets is below the annular line (LV side). 'Bowing' occurs when there is normal coaptation, but the body of the valve leaflet is redundant and enlarged and arcs into the left atrium during systole. Prolapse occurs when the coaptation point of one or more of the leaflet scallops occurs above the annular line (LA side). MV prolapse or Barlow's syndrome is associated with normal valve leaflets. Prolapse-associated MR and myxomatous disease show abnormal leaflet morphology (described earlier) and the tricuspid or aortic valves may be also affected.

Flail segments occur when there is an elongated or ruptured chorda with one leaflet edge extending above the other into the LA. The edge of the flail leaflet points into the atrium during systole, with an eccentric colour flow jet directed away from the flail over the atrial side of the other leaflet. Patients with flail segments present with severe MR. Rarely, a papillary muscle head may be attached to the chords of a flail segment and observed in the LA during systole. This is secondary to acute myocardial infarction with acute severe MR with normal-sized LA and LV.

Systolic motion of the anterior mitral valve leaflet (SAM) may cause MR. High-velocity flow in the LVOT creates a Venturi effect that moves the MV coaptation point anteriorly into the LVOT until the anterior mitral valve leaflet (AMVL) is sucked away from the posterior mitral valve leaflet (PMVL) late in systole, causing an eccentric jet of MR across the PMVL. This may occur with subvalvular ridges or hypertrophic obstructive cardiomyopathy.

Subvalvular attachments (chordae, papillary muscles and the LV wall): Chordae can restrict the valve leaflets from closing during systole if they are shortened and thickened as in rheumatic heart disease, or if they are being pulled apically during systole because of ischaemic left ventricular dyskinesis or abnormal orientation of the papillary muscles as in cardiomyopathy. Acute LV volume overload may result in a central jet of MR because of displacement of the subvalvular attachments. Ventricular wall dysfunction during acute myocardial ischaemia can produce MR by a similar mechanism.

The chordae in myxomatous degeneration may be elongated and prolapse or rupture, creating flail segments.

Qualitative markers of MR severity are chamber enlargement and PV flow reversal. Quantitative markers include jet area, effective regurgitant orifice (ERO), regurgitant volume (RegV), regurgitant fraction (RF), and vena contracta width (VCW) (Table 10.4).

Table 10.4 Quantification of mitral regurgitation

Grade	ERO (mm^2)	Jet area/LA area (%)	RegV (mL)	RF (%)	VCW (cm)
Normal			<5	<10	
Mild	<20	<20		20–30	<0.3
Moderate	20–29	20–40		30–50	0.3–0.7
Severe	>40	>40	>60	>50	>0.7

Tricuspid valve

Tricuspid stenosis

Stenosis may be a result of rheumatic heart disease with fusion of leaflets, or retracted cusps and subvalvular apparatus. Carcinoid may cause either regurgitation or stenosis of the pulmonary or tricuspid valves. Right atrial thrombus and masses may obstruct the TV and cause stenosis.

Tricuspid regurgitation

Normal leaflets: Annular dilatation caused by distension of the RA or RV, secondary to left heart failure, primary pulmonary hypertension, or left-to-right shunts.

Abnormal valve with leaflet destruction: Systemic lupus erythematosus (SLE) induced endocarditis or endocarditis in intravenous drug users may cause TR. Pacemakers or cardiac catheters may damage the valve, resulting in TR.

Abnormal valve with leaflet restriction: In 20% of cases of tricuspid valve disease the cause is rheumatic (predominantly TR). Commissural fusion is difficult to detect. Carcinoid results in shortened, thickened and stiff valve leaflets with incomplete coaptation causing TR in 90% of cases, and less commonly TS. Dietary- and drug-induced valvulitis can produce a similar picture to carcinoid. Carcinoid occurs in 1/75 000 with 90% arising from the GI tract and 50% of patients develop carcinoid syndrome, in which tryptophan is converted by the tumour to 5HT, histamine, tachykinins and prostaglandins, causing flushing, diarrhoea, and bronchoconstriction, and in 50% of cases there is cardiac pathology, particularly if there are hepatic metastases. The TV is involved in 97% and the PV in 88% of cases. Fibrous plaques appear as thickened echodense areas on the valve leaflets, subvalvular apparatus, cardiac chambers and the IVC. Calcification usually does not occur. CW Doppler of the TR shows a dagger-shaped regurgitant jet with a high peak pressure and rapid decline. Left-sided involvement of the MV occurs in 7% because of a patent foramen ovale, or extensive liver or bronchial metastases.

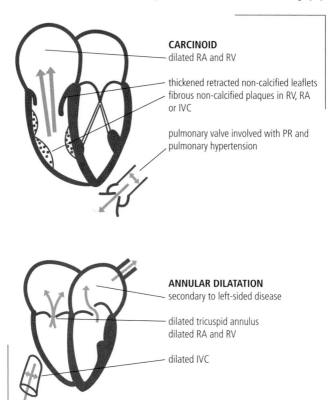

CARCINOID
— dilated RA and RV

thickened retracted non-calcified leaflets
fibrous non-calcified plaques in RV, RA
or IVC

pulmonary valve involved with PR and
pulmonary hypertension

ANNULAR DILATATION
— secondary to left-sided disease

— dilated tricuspid annulus
dilated RA and RV

— dilated IVC

Figure 10.6 Tricuspid regurgitation

Ebstein's anomaly: As shown in Figure 10.7, the leaflets are inserted lower into the RV, atrialising part of the RV. There is a restricted, redundant, sail-like anterosuperior leaflet with chords attaching directly to the free RV wall.

The increased stroke volume across the TV causes dilatation of the RV and RA and paradoxical movement of the interventricular septum towards the RV during systole. Flow reversal may be detected in the first hepatic vein (Figure 10.8).

Indications for tricuspid repair include severity, indexed size of the annulus >2.1 cm²/m², RF >25% and reduced RV function. Repair is

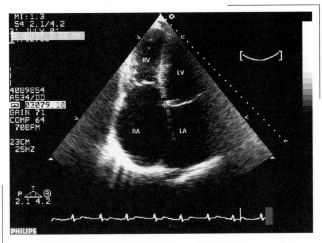

Figure 10.7 Ebstein's anomaly showing apical displacement of the tricuspid valve leaflets (TTE Ap4ch)

with a ring or suture annuloplasty. If valve replacement is required, a bioprosthesis is used because it has greater durability in the right heart than in the left.

Pulmonary valve

Pulmonary stenosis
Pulmonary stenosis (PS) is rare and usually the result of congenital PS persisting into adult life, or carcinoid syndrome. Assessment is usually with pressure gradients.

Pulmonary regurgitation
Mild pulmonary regurgitation (PR) may be a normal finding; however, severe PR may occur in congenital disease with small, thickened leaflets. Endocarditis, carcinoid, and myxomatous degeneration represent acquired abnormalities. Leaflet morphology indicates aetiology, with redundant leaflets being consistent with myxomatous change and thick, shortened, immobile leaflets with carcinoid. The PV is involved in 88% of carcinoid cardiac abnormalities, with PR in 81% and PS in 53%. Both may worsen the TR.

(a)
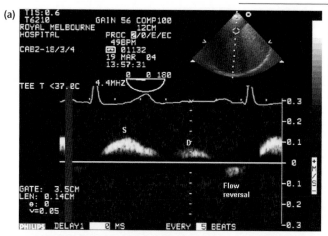

(b)
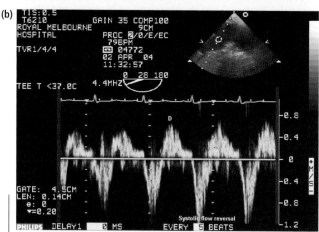

Figure 10.8 Hepatic vein Doppler showing (a) normal, larger S systolic wave, smaller D diastolic wave and normal retrograde flow. (b) Systolic flow reversal consistent with significant TR

Evaluation of valvular stenosis

Quantification is either via gradients or valve area.

Assessment of gradients

Mean pressure gradients and peak pressure gradients have been described in Chapter 7. Gradients are directly proportional to SV and CO, so the degree of stenosis may be underestimated if there is poor LV function. Prosthetic valves have high-flow jets, in which case mean gradient should be used.

Assessment of valve area

Area can be calculated by pressure half-time (PHT), continuity equation or proximal isovelocity surface area (PISA) methods. The continuity equation is not affected by either SV or CO.

Pressure half-time: PHT is used to calculate the MVA in MS. In response to a stenotic MV the high LAP gives rise to a greater peak velocity. Emptying of the LA into the LV takes longer and the velocity of the blood flow slowly drops as the pressure differential slowly falls. This is measured as the deceleration time (DT) of the E wave. The time taken for the LA–LV pressure difference to drop from its peak to half is the PHT, which is related to DT:

$$PHT = 0.29 \times DT$$

DT and PHT are directly related to MVA:

$$MVA\ (cm^2) = 220/PHT\ (ms) = 759/DT\ (ms)$$

The constant '220' was empirically derived in patients with MVA close to 1 cm^3 and is more accurate for valve areas close to this figure than for normal valves.

PHT is inaccurate when a change in LV compliance contributes to reducing the flow across the MV, such as in severe AR.

Continuity equation: Calculation of MVA using the continuity equation has been described in Chapter 7. In patients with a low CO, dobutamine or exercise can be used to maximise valve opening. The dimensionless index (LVOT$_{VTI}$/AV$_{VTI}$ ratio) is a flow-independent

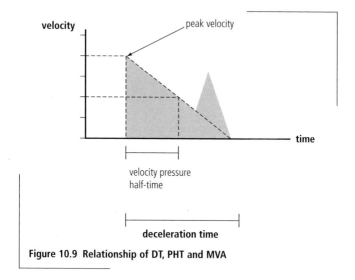

Figure 10.9 Relationship of DT, PHT and MVA

measure of the severity of AS, but is subject to the same limitations as those that may be encountered with the continuity equation. A value <0.25 for native aortic valves is indicative of severe AS.

Proximal isovelocity surface area: PISA is a further application of the continuity equation that makes use of the facts that flow proximal to a stenosis converges towards the stenosis and that points of equal flow form concentric hemispheres about the stenosis. Adjusting the Nyquist limit defines a hemisphere in which flow displays aliasing (Figure 10.10). The flow is the Nyquist flow (V_n) at this point. The area of this hemisphere ($2\pi r^2$) can be determined by measuring its radius with the stenosis at its centre. Peak velocity through the stenosis is measured (V_{MS}). If the valve leaflets funnel into the stenosis, the area of the hemisphere is reduced. The angle between the leaflets (θ) can be used as a correction factor ($\theta/180$).

$$\text{MVA} = \frac{2\pi r^2 \times V_n}{V_{MS}} \times \frac{\theta}{180}$$

PISA is used to estimate the valve area of stenotic mitral and tricuspid valves, and the ERO in regurgitant valve lesions.

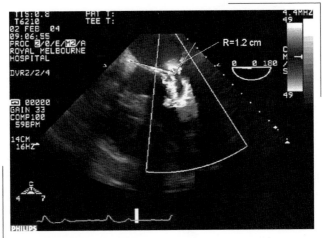

Figure 10.10 PISA hemisphere

Evaluation of valvular regurgitation

Forward flow across a regurgitant valve increases as the valve becomes more regurgitant. Stroke volume increases the VTI and peak velocity. A dense CW signal and 'V-shaped' envelope of the regurgitant jet also indirectly indicate the severity of regurgitation.

In MR the LV afterload is reduced because of ejection into the low pressure LA, so LV systolic function appears better than it really is. Normal LV function will appear as hyperdynamic, which becomes important when MR is secondary to a dilated cardiomyopathy or an ischaemic left ventricle, because true systolic function is often substantially worse than it appears.

Flow reversal seen in the pulmonary veins during systole is associated with severe MR. Flow reversal is also seen in the first hepatic vein in TR and in the upper descending aorta throughout diastole with severe AR (holodiastolic flow).

Quantification

Regurgitant jet: Jet length and area are useful only for mild or very severe MR. Central jets entrain blood; eccentric jets appear smaller in volume because of the coanda effect and are often graded up.

Regurgitant jet diameter compared with the diameter of the LVOT: Used to quantify AR.

Regurgitant volume and fraction: This is the fraction of blood that is returned to the chamber after systole. The forward SV across a regurgitant valve (SVr) is equal to the forward SV across a non-regurgitant valve (SVn) plus the regurgitant volume (RegV).

$$RF = \frac{RegV}{SVr} \times 100\%$$

Effective regurgitant orifice: ERO is calculated using the regurgitant volume as calculated above or with PISA, but angle corrections are not usually applied for MR. A 3D representation of the regurgitant orifice area in real time for the duration of MR is a future method of assessment.

$$ERO = 2\pi r^2 \times Vn/Vregurg_{max}$$

Pressure half-time: The Doppler flow pattern of the regurgitant jet reflects the pressure differential between the aortic root and the LV: the faster the two equalise, the quicker the flow returns to baseline. A short PHT reflects a higher grade of AR.

Vena contracta width: VCW is the smallest width of a regurgitant jet and its measurement has been validated for mild and severe MR and for eccentric jets.

Evaluation of prosthetic valves

Prosthetic valves are either mechanical or bioprosthetic. The types of mechanical valves are bileaflet, single tilting disc, or caged ball. Biological valves are stented heterografts, such as porcine or bovine pericardium, stentless heterografts, homografts from human cadavers (allograft) or autografts (e.g. the Ross procedure in which a PV is transplanted to the aortic position and a pulmonary homograft is used).

Mechanical valves are durable, but have higher incidence of thromboembolism and anticoagulant bleeding complications, whereas biological valves have lower thrombotic and bleeding concerns but reduced durability.

Mechanical valves

Thromboembolism with mechanical valves has a mortality of 0.2% and morbidity of 1–2% per patient year. Thromboembolic events occur more frequently for mitral than aortic mechanical valves, and are more likely with the caged ball and tilting disc types than with bileaflet valves.

Bileaflet valve: The most common mechanical valve is the bileaflet type, which consists of a pyrolytic carbon ring and semicircular leaflets that open to 85° and close to 25° to the plane of the horizontal ring. When imaging with CFD parallel to the hinge points there is acoustic shadowing from the ring, reverberation artifact from the leaflets below the valve, and an inverted V-shaped 'washing jet' arising from the hinge points. When imaging at 90° to the line of the hinge points, the leaflets open to 85° below the ring and smaller V-shaped 'washing jets' arise from each hinge point. These washing jets prevent clot formation of the MV hinges. Sometimes a third central jet can be seen. Prior to separating from bypass one leaflet is kept open by a LV vent or is caught up in the subvalvular apparatus until the LV is distended, in order to aid de-airing. CW exhibits bright vertical line clicks of opening and closure.

There is a closure jet of regurgitation that is separate to the washing jets. The combination of leakage and the washing jets usually comprises only 10% of forward flow, but can increase to 30% with tachycardia or low CO.

Single tilting disc (Bjork Shiley) valves: This type of valve opens to 75° in the aortic position and 70° in the mitral position. There may be small peripheral regurgitant jets alone or in combination with a prominent central jet. Fracture of the strut housing was an early problem that led to development of monostrut designs.

Caged ball (Starr Edwards) valve: The S-E valve has two U-shaped arches at right-angles that house a silicone ball with no MR in the closed position. It has a high profile; that is, the arches intrude into the LVOT.

Bioprosthetic valves

Bioprosthetic valves tend to degenerate after 10–15 years (earlier in the mitral than in the aortic area and earlier in younger patients) and failure is caused by high shearing forces on the valve leaflets. Larger valves are at greater risk, as are patients who are susceptible to calcification, such as in chronic renal failure or familial hyperlipidaemia. Despite this, there has been an apparent increase in the use of bioprosthetic valves because of the increased age of patients coming to surgery, the improved durability of the valves, and identification of patients under 70 years of age who have reduced longevity because of comorbidity and reduced morbidity with a second operation.

These valves are trileaflet with trivial central regurgitation, and in larger valves commissural regurgitant jets may be seen. The sewing ring impacts upon the valve area, so smaller diameter valves are mildly stenotic. Stentless valves may be chosen for patients with a small aortic annulus because the effective orifice is 10% greater than with the corresponding stented valve. Although greater durability is stated, they require a longer cardiopulmonary bypass time because of the extensive suture line.

The goals of the Ross procedure are to supply low gradients, durability and no need for anticoagulation, and it is performed in young patients with AS or AR.

Follow-up of prosthetic valves

Peak velocity, peak and mean gradients, and valve areas have been used to follow valve function (Table 10.5). Peak velocity is high in bileaflet mechanical valves because of the high turbulent flow through

Table 10.5 Follow-up of prosthetic valves

St Jude prosthesis	Peak gradient (mmHg)	Mean gradient (mmHg)
19 mm aortic	31.2 ± 17.3	22.2 ± 11
21 mm	30 ± 5.7	14.4 ± 5
23 mm	23.2 ± 11.5	10.8 ± 6
25 mm	19.8 ± 8.2	11 ± 6
27 mm mitral	10.11 ± 3.43	5 ± 2
29 mm	9.9 ± 4.49	2.71 ± 1.36

the central portion of the valve. Estimates of area and peak gradient using peak velocity will underestimate the valve area and overestimate peak gradient. Mean velocity is also increased, but closer to the true mean gradient.

Areas calculated by the continuity equation are accurate; however, PHT overestimates it for mechanical valves compared with bioprosthetic valves because of the higher peak velocities of these valves.

Complications with prosthetic valves

Imaging can be difficult when there is a prosthetic valve because of the acoustic shadowing from the valve struts and ring and reverberation from the leaflets. The aortic annulus and LVOT are difficult to image in the TOE MO AV LAX and SAX views because of interference from the sewing ring, but can be seen in the deep TG LAX AV view. However, the latter view is compromised when there is double valve replacement, with the MV obscuring the AV.

Thromboembolism and bleeding: Vascular complications represent 75% and 50% of the complications with mechanical and bioprosthetic valves, respectively. Direct visualisation of thrombus is hard because of the rings and struts. Partial immobility of a valve leaflet and a new stenosis are indirect indications of a thrombus. TOE can document regression of thrombus after thrombolytic therapy.

Stenosis by pannus ingrowth: Degenerative change in the vessel wall causes progressive calcification and fibrous ingrowth (pannus) over the ring, impeding the orifice and resulting in MS or AS. Trends in velocity and gradients are used to follow the development of stenosis.

Paravalvular leak: Ring dehiscence may occur early because of suture failure, late because of degenerative calcification, or be related to endocarditis. A regurgitant jet is seen outside the bright ring image and is confirmed in two views. Small jets seen around the ring sutures immediately after separation from cardiopulmonary bypass are not pathological and disappear after reversal of heparin.

Valve failure: This is a rare but catastrophic event. Strut breakage may occur in single-disc valves, leaflets may become fixed open or closed in bileaflet valves and the cage may dehisce from the sewing ring in caged ball valves.

Endocarditis

Endocarditis in patients with prosthetic valves has a high mortality. Infected mechanical valves usually have an associated abscess, whereas bioprosthetic valves become stenotic or regurgitant because of valve destruction. Vegetations are not the primary feature and are smaller than in native valves, with size not predictive of embolisation potential. Vegetations may appear as a thickening or irregularity on the valve sewing ring, but could also be pannus or thrombus. Strands on a mitral prosthesis may represent false-positive findings. Prosthetic aortic vegetations have a higher paravalvular abscess rate (6%) and require surgical intervention. Prosthetic valve endocarditic embolisation occurs in 13–40% of cases, particularly from the MV.

Echocardiographic assessment of infective endocarditis

Echocardiography has become pivotal in the diagnosis of infective endocarditis. Dukes established major and minor criteria from the clinical, microbiological and echocardiographic features, with diagnosis requiring two major, or one major and three minor, criteria. The major echocardiographic criteria are:

- Vegetations—defined as echodense masses implanted in the valve or mural endocardium in the trajectory of a regurgitant jet or implanted in prosthetic material with no alternative anatomical explanation
- Abscess
- New dehiscence of a valvular prosthesis.

Although other abnormal echocardiographic findings are regarded as minor criteria, other studies have suggested they be included as major criteria because of improved 2D resolution. Original minor criteria included valvular perforation, nodular thickening and non-mobile masses.

Aseptic vegetations may occur in SLE and antiphospholipid syndrome, such as Libman-Sacks endocarditis or marantic endocarditis.

Cardiac complications of infective endocarditis

- Valvular perforation
- Perivalvar abscess—seen as an echolucent area and occurs in 37% of cases, with a mortality of 40–90%. It usually forms

in the membranous septum, which is the weakest portion of the septum. Abscess is easier to see in the aortic area

- Mycotic aneurysm and intracardiac fistula
- Aortic root abscess/pseudoaneurysm—may rupture into the adjacent RA and LA.

Chapter 11

Problems with great vessels

David Andrews

Learning objectives

1. Understand the limitations of echocardiography in diagnosing common aortic pathology.
2. Understand the role of intraoperative epiaortic ultrasound.

Evaluation of the great vessels

Thoracic aorta

The thoracic aorta can be divided into three sections—the ascending aorta, the aortic arch and the descending thoracic aorta. There are six imaging planes required to interrogate the thoracic aorta by TOE (see Figures 5.3, 5.5):

1. Mid-oesophageal ascending aorta short axis (MO asc. aorta SAX)
2. Mid-oesophageal ascending aorta long axis (MO asc. aorta LAX)
3. Upper oesophageal aortic arch short axis (UO aortic arch SAX)
4. Upper oesophageal aortic arch long axis (UO aortic arch LAX)
5. Descending aorta short axis (MO desc. aorta SAX)
6. Descending aorta long axis (MO desc. aorta LAX)

Limitations: The anatomic limitation is that the relationship of the trachea to the ascending thoracic aorta results in an air interface between the TOE transducer and the aorta, which limits the operator's ability to fully interrogate the region that includes the distal ascending aorta and proximal aortic arch. The use of TOE alone in the assessment of the ascending thoracic aorta is subject to imaging artifacts caused by a lack of both specificity and sensitivity. Lack of specificity leads to linear artifacts being seen when interrogating the thoracic aorta with TOE and these have been described in up to 44–55% of cases of aortic dissection. They are most commonly caused by reverberation, resulting in multiple reflection pathways when the ultrasound beam strikes an interface where large impedance mismatches occur between tissues, particularly if the interface is oriented perpendicular to the ultrasound beam. With regard to sensitivity, many studies have shown that epiaortic ultrasound is more sensitive than TOE in identifying atheroma in the ascending aorta and one in particular showed that when comparing epiaortic ultrasound with TOE in cardiac surgical patients, TOE failed to identify lesions that were consistently larger than 4 mm in size in the middle and distal segments of the ascending aorta.

Therefore, the use of epiaortic ultrasound in combination with TOE during cardiac surgery enables an overall greater assessment of the thoracic aorta. The epiaortic ultrasound transducers may be either linear or phased array. Phased array probes have a small footprint, with easy access and approximation to the ascending aorta, but are limited by lateral resolution quality and crowding of the near-field image. A standoff (plastic spacing device) may be required between the aorta and transducer to prevent crowding of the near-field image. The linear array transducers (although they have a larger footprint that can impede approximation to the vessel wall) offer excellent lateral resolution, and often do not require a standoff. It is important to use a high-frequency transducer (>8 MHz) to provide good resolution. Images of the thoracic aorta can be obtained using TTE, but the resolution is poor because of the low-frequency transducer. Useful Doppler information may be obtained.

Pulmonary artery

The interrogation of the main, left and right PA with TOE is possible using the following imaging planes (see Figure 5.3):

1. Mid-oesophageal right ventricular inflow-outflow (MO RV inflow–outflow)
2. Mid-oesophageal ascending aorta short axis (MO asc. aorta SAX)

3. Mid-oesophageal ascending aorta long axis (MO asc. aorta LAX)
4. Upper oesophageal aortic arch short axis (UO aortic arch SAX)

Aortic dilatation: A thoracic aortic aneurysm is considered to be present when there is localised dilatation of the aorta greater than 1.5-fold the expected normal values, which are shown in Table 11.1.

Table 11.1 Thoracic aorta diameters for TOE and epiaortic ultrasound

Site	Diameter (cm)
Aortic annulus	1.4–2.6
Trans-sinus	2.1–3.5
Sino-tubular junction	1.7–3.4
Ascending aorta	2.1–3.4
Aortic arch	2.0–3.6

Aortic dissection: Aortic dissection (AD) is described by either the DeBakey or Stanford classification system (Figure 11.1). Both DeBakey types I and II have the AD membrane originating in the ascending aorta. The DeBakey type I dissection extends around to involve the descending thoracic aorta whereas in type II the dissection is localised to the ascending aorta. DeBakey type III has the AD membrane originating in the descending thoracic aorta, distal to the origin of the left subclavian artery. The Stanford system divides AD into two types, A and B, depending on which part of the aorta is involved regardless of the origin of the dissection membrane. Stanford type A involves the ascending aorta and type B is localised to the descending thoracic aorta. It is the more frequently used classification nomenclature because the treatment of each type is very different: type A requires immediate surgical intervention whereas type B can be treated conservatively.

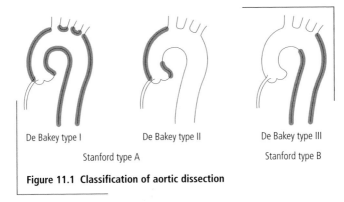

De Bakey type I De Bakey type II De Bakey type III

Stanford type A Stanford type B

Figure 11.1 Classification of aortic dissection

Aortic dissection in the emergency department

Acute AD is a life-threatening condition and prompt diagnosis is essential for successful management. The imaging modalities available include retrograde aortography, contrast-enhanced computed tomography (CTA), magnetic resonance imaging (MRI) and TOE. Of these, aortography had long been considered the gold standard in diagnosing AD, but has now ceased to be the reference technique because it is limited in cases of false-lumen thrombosis and acute aortic syndrome (see later). The advent of high-resolution MRI has resulted in diagnostic sensitivities and specificities uniformly approaching 100% and it has become the imaging modality of first choice for AD. However, MRI is not always practical. TOE compares favourably to MRI in the diagnosis of AD and performs better than TTE, CTA or aortography. In addition, TOE is expedient, minimally invasive, requires no contrast, can be performed at the patient's bedside and provides a dynamic assessment of the cardiovascular system. Demonstration of an aortic intimal flap or membrane that divides the aorta into two lumina, true and false, forms the basis of echocardiographic diagnosis of AD. Ranges for sensitivity (97–100%), specificity (68–100%), positive-predictive (98–100%) and negative-predictive (96–99%) values for TOE have been reported from multiple studies of the diagnosis of AD.

Limitations: The main diagnostic limitation of TOE is a small type A dissection localised to the ascending aorta. The presence of an intraluminal linear image is not sufficient to make the diagnosis of AD and in this situation it is considered that the diagnosis of type A dissection should only be accepted when other accompanying findings, such as aortic insufficiency, intimal tear, intraluminal thrombosis or pericardial effusion, are present.

Therefore, when presented with a patient with suspected AD in the ED, a non-invasive diagnostic strategy using MRI in the haemodynamically stable patient or TOE in the unstable patient is considered the optimal approach in detecting acute thoracic AD.

Repair of aortic dissection or aneurysm

The combination of TOE and epiaortic ultrasound can be used intraoperatively and is a powerful aid in the decision making for surgical intervention in AD or aneurysm repair. Both modalities have a role in delineating aortic wall pathology, in particular localising intramural haematoma and atheroma, locating dissection membranes, and assessing directional blood flow beneath membranes and false lumens. Additionally, TOE is useful in the dynamic interrogation of the aortic valve and pericardium with respect to associated aortic insufficiency or pericardial tamponade. Furthermore, TOE can be used in the therapeutic decision-making and evaluation of other blood vessels; for example, AD or aneurysm that extends and involves the origin of the carotid and subclavian arteries, and the presence of ventricular wall motion abnormalities may indicate that the coronary arteries are affected by the AD. Involvement of the coronary arteries is considered to occur in 10–15% of cases of acute AD, with the right coronary artery most frequently affected. When the aortic arch is involved with AD it is important to ascertain the origin of the supra-aortic vessels from the true or false aortic lumen: a false lumen is normally larger and has less flow than the true lumen. However, sometimes it can be difficult to determine, in which case M-mode ultrasound can be used to show intimal movement towards the false lumen at the start of systole because of the expansion of the true aortic lumen.

Endovascular repair of the aorta is an alternative to open repair and TOE is used to identify the extent of the aneurysm or dissection and guide the placement of the wire and stent in combination with radiological techniques. CFD can supplement angiography to detect flow within the aneurysmal sac after stent placement, as well as identifying any endoleaks.

Secondary findings: (1) Secondary tears: CFD may indicate multiple communications between the true and false lumina. Multiple fenestrations have been detected in up to 35% of ascending AD and up to 70% of descending thoracic AD. (2) False-lumen thrombus: formation of a false-lumen thrombus depends on the type of dissection and its location. TOE has an accuracy of 90%, compared with 65% for aortography, in detecting false-lumen thrombus. Thrombus formation in the false lumen is a positive prognostic finding.

Other aortic pathology

Acute aortic syndrome
Processes such as intramural haematoma and penetrating atherosclerotic ulcers are being increasingly recognised as additional causes of acute chest pain. The sensitivity and specificity of TOE in diagnosing these pathologies has not been reported, and therefore should be confirmed with other diagnostic techniques, such as MRI or epiaortic ultrasound, if found at the time of surgery. Treatment for all three conditions has thus far been dictated by location (as for AD).

Diagnosis of intramural haematoma by TOE is made when a circular or semilunar image, which may contain layers of heterogeneous echogenicity, surrounds or closely approximates the aortic wall. Subgroups of type A intramural haematoma may be treated medically with good outcomes.

Diagnosis and differentiation of penetrating atherosclerotic ulcers with TOE can be more difficult. The presence of saccular protrusions outside the profile of the aorta may be hard to visualise with TOE. Colour Doppler and epiaortic ultrasound may assist if the lesion is accessible.

Traumatic aortic disruption
Immediate surgical intervention is required, but the diagnosis of aortic rupture may be difficult to make with TOE. Pericardial or pleural effusions are suspicious of aortic transection. Increased distance between the oesophagus and LA or descending thoracic aorta is a subtle sign. CFD interrogation may help in the diagnosis.

Aortic coarctation

Re-coarctaton of the aorta can occur in 10% of individuals with the disease. It is commonly seen with TOE just distal to the left subclavian artery origin.

Patent ductus arteriosus

PDA is rarely seen in adults and difficult to image with TOE. If present, high-velocity aliased flow can be seen in the left or main PA when using CFD.

Assessment of atheroma with epiaortic ultrasound

Both the severity and location of atheromatous disease in the ascending aorta are independent risk factors for postoperative ischaemic cerebral injury following cardiac surgery. Atheroma of the aorta can be classified according to the width of intimal thickening and the complexity of the atheroma: normal <2 mm thick, mild 2–4 mm or moderate >4 mm with flat plaque; severe >4 mm and complex ('hills and valleys' appearance) or mobile plaque. Disease in the proximal third and mid-lateral segments of the ascending aorta is associated with a higher incidence of postoperative stroke, irrespective of the extent of the disease. However, even intimal thickening >2 mm (grade II–III disease) of the ascending aorta and aortic arch has been shown to contribute to stroke after cardiac surgery. Intraoperative epiaortic ultrasound has a high sensitivity and specificity for detecting aortic atheroma and has become the modality of choice for detecting plaque within the aorta during cardiac surgery because it is superior to either TOE or aortic palpation for this purpose. Moreover, detection of atheroma in the descending thoracic aorta by TOE has been shown to be a surrogate indicator of ascending aortic atheroma and correlates with the risk of stroke following cardiac surgery. Recently, 3D epiaortic ultrasound has been shown to be superior to any 2D imaging modality in identifying, localising, and defining the true extent of plaque in the aorta.

Assessment of pulmonary embolism

Pulmonary embolism (PE) can occur in many postoperative scenarios and in some cases is associated with significant morbidity and mortality. PE is usually diagnosed by pulmonary angiography or CTA, spiral CT or ventilation-perfusion scintigraphy; however, in an unstable patient it may not be possible to undertake these investigations. Unfortunately, TOE is not a reliable technique for directly visualising PE in the intraoperative setting of pulmonary embolectomy. Furthermore, it is least sensitive for directly visualising PE in the left PA because thrombo-emboli located in this region may be obscured by the interposition of the left main bronchus anterior to the oesophagus, resulting in a reduction in diagnostic image quality. However, TOE is more helpful in detecting indirect signs and consequences of PA obstruction. There is a high incidence of RV dysfunction and dilatation, TR and leftward bowing of the interatrial septum accompanying haemodynamically significant PE and these can be easily detected with TOE.

Chapter 12

Problems with pericardium and pleura

Reny Segal

Learning objectives
1. Understand the role of echocardiography in the assessment of pericardial and pleural disease.
2. Understand the role of echocardiography in pericardial tamponade.
3. Understand the limitations and alternative approaches to echocardiography.

Assessment of pericardial and pleural disease

Echocardiography is used in numerous sub-specialties, such as cardiology, cardiothoracic anaesthesia, emergency medicine, trauma medicine and intensive care, and emerging in the field of non-cardiac anaesthesia. However, it is interesting to remember that echocardiography originally gained attention for its ability to detect pericardial effusion. So, in this chapter the 'humble' pericardium will be reviewed, as will the disease states that affect it and thus influence the cardiac chambers contained within its not so compliant vault. The differentiation between pleural and pericardial effusion using echocardiography will also be addressed.

Pericardial anatomy

During development, the heart invaginates into a potential cavity called the pericardial space. On the outside of this potential cavity is the thin and fibrous parietal pericardium, which is in close contact with both the pleura laterally and diaphragm inferiorly, and when the pericardium is described, it refers to this parietal layer. On the inside is the visceral pericardium, which is continuous with the cardiac surface/epicardium and cannot be separated. The pericardial space (between the two layers) contains a small quantity of serous fluid (5–10 mL) that acts as a lubricant.

The pericardium is attached posteriorly to the pulmonary veins and the venae cava and superiorly to the great arteries. It is these attachments that give rise to two blind-ending pouches: the oblique and transverse sinuses (Figure 12.1). Again, as with the pericardial space, these sinuses are potential spaces that become prominent on echocardiography only when fluid (or cysts, clots or fatty infiltration) is present.

Pericardial physiology

This topic is open to debate that is beyond the scope of this chapter. Some believe that the pericardium limits cardiac distension, modulates intracavity pressures and mediates ventricular coupling. Others believe that the pericardium has no significant haemodynamic function at all and attains its importance only in disease.

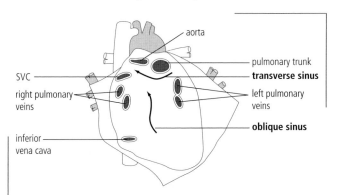

Figure 12.1 Pericardial cavity (posterior surface) demonstrating transverse and oblique sinuses

Normal pericardium on echocardiography: The normal pericardium will be visible on most echocardiography views (see Chapters 5 and 6) as a single, thin echogenic structure that is more prominent posteriorly.

With pericardial inflammation (as in pericarditis), there may be a degree of pericardial thickening that may be visible on 2D and M-mode imaging and there may be an associated pericardial effusion. However, the pericardium is normally the most echogenic structure anyway and distinguishing normal from thickened pericardium is not easy. Furthermore, the absence of an effusion does not exclude the diagnosis of pericarditis. Pericarditis is not easily diagnosed with echocardiography alone.

Pericardial effusion

Definition
A pericardial effusion is the presence or accumulation of an abnormal quantity of fluid in the pericardial space (i.e. >5–10 mL). However, the presence of a pericardial effusion does not in itself imply haemodynamic changes or physiologic compromise.

Causes
There are six main causes of pericardial effusion.
1. Infectious
   - Bacterial
   - Viral
   - Tuberculous
2. Malignant
   - Primary cardiac
   - Contiguous (lung, breast)
   - Metastatic (melanoma, lymphatic)
3. Inflammatory
   - Post cardiac surgery
   - Post myocardial infarct (Dressler's syndrome)
   - Collagen disease
   - Renal failure (uraemia)
4. Cardiac (pericardiac space communications)
   - Chest trauma
   - LV rupture post infarction
   - Post-catheter procedures (interventional cardiology)

5. Idiopathic
6. 'Other'
   - Asbestosis
   - Radiation

Echocardiographic diagnosis

It is important to distinguish pericardial fluid from pericardial tamponade because there may be a large pericardial effusion with no haemodynamic compromise whatsoever or, conversely, a small pericardial effusion with significant compromise.

Useful views for interrogating pericardial effusions

TOE (Figure 12.2a)
- MO 4-chamber view
- TG SAX mid-papillary view

TTE (Figure 12.2b)
- Subcostal 4-chamber view
- PLAX view
- Parasternal SAX LV views
- Apical 4-chamber view

Pericardial effusion presents as:
- echolucent space adjacent to the cardiac structures: the larger this space, the larger the effusion
- symmetrical (anterior and posterior) in the absence of pericardial disease or surgery
- a collection large enough to give the appearance of a 'swinging' heart

M-mode is also useful for examining a pericardial effusion. The interrogating beam, aligned perpendicularly in the TG MID SAX (TOE) or parasternal LAX or SAX views (TTE), will show separation between the flat, posterior pericardial echo reflection and the moving epicardial echo in both systole and diastole.

Quantifying the size of the effusion: With one echo caliper placed on the epicardium and the other on the parietal pericardium, the effusion (space) is small (<0.5 cm), moderate (0.5–2.0 cm) or large (>2.0 cm). These sizes are arbitrary and in isolation cannot determine haemodynamic significance.

(a)
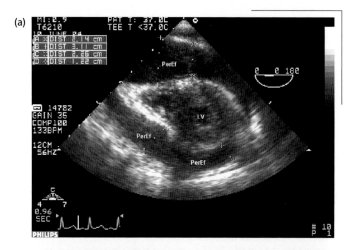

(b)
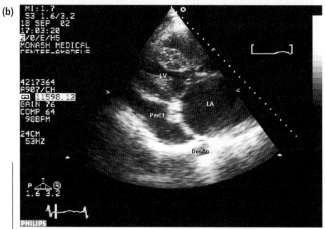

Figure 12.2 Pericardial effusion. (a) TOE TG mid SAX, (b) TTE PLAX

Is it pericardial or pleural fluid?
- First, look for the echogenic pericardium—this is your anchor point.
- In the TOE views (MO 4-chamber, TG mid SAX) or TTE view (PLAX) any fluid between the pericardium and the heart is pericardial fluid (Figure 12.3).
- An isolated free space, superior to the RA, is usually pleural fluid.

Identify the descending aorta
- Pleural effusion will extend *posterolateral* to the descending aorta.
- Pericardial effusion will extend *anterior* to the descending aorta.
- The space between the LA and the descending aorta will be splayed by a pericardial effusion, but not by a left pleural effusion.

Pericardial tamponade

Most texts refer to tamponade physiology, which is quite correct and explains the whole concept. The term 'tamponade' refers to the physiological changes associated with an increase in the pericardial fluid, causing increased pressure when the pericardium has reached its limit of stretch. This concept can be demonstrated on the pressure–volume (compliance) curve (Figure 12.4).

A key factor in tamponade is time, which should be added to the pressure–volume relationship. Rapidly forming collections will exceed pericardial stretch at a relatively low volume, resulting in a steeply rising intrapericardial pressure that is transmitted to the cardiac chambers and causes haemodynamic compromise.

In contrast, collections that form slowly (weeks to months) enable the pericardium to stretch and compensatory mechanisms to occur. Much higher volumes will be tolerated before the pericardial stretch limit is breached and the rapid rise in pressure is demonstrated on the compliance curve (i.e. critical tamponade). It is not unusual to drain 1000 mL from a slowly accumulating pericardial effusion without much haemodynamic compromise prior to a procedure.

(a)

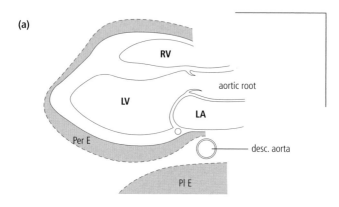

(b)

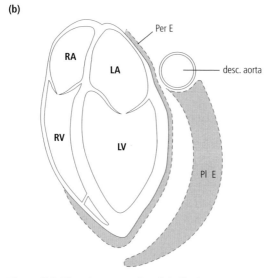

Figure 12.3 Pleural versus pericardial effusion. (a) TTE PLAX view: fluid anterior to the descending aorta is pericardial (Per E), whereas fluid posterior to the vessel is pleural (Pl E). (b) TOE MO 4-chamber view shows fluid in the pleural space as a 'tiger claw' pointing towards the left of the screen

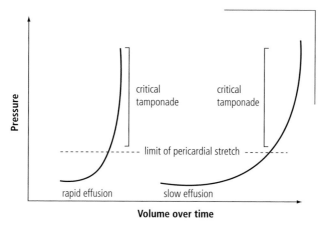

Figure 12.4 Pressure–volume (compliance) curve

Clinical features of acute tamponade

You might, in all fairness, ask 'Why do the clinical features of tamponade appear in an echocardiography book?' The rational is that tamponade is both a clinical and a haemodynamic diagnosis, and not simply an echocardiographic one.

1. Low cardiac output
   - Hypotension
   - Tachycardia
   - Poor peripheral perfusion
   - Altered sensorium (if very severe)
2. Elevated jugular venous pressure
3. Pulsus paradoxus
4. Muffled heart sounds (non-specific)

In a patient with suspected clinical tamponade, the presence on echocardiography of a pericardial effusion confirms the diagnosis. Conversely, the lack of effusion excludes this diagnosis.

Pulsus paradoxus is an exaggerated response (>10–15 mmHg) to the normal physiological process of a decrease in systolic blood pressure during inspiration. The importance of pulsus paradoxus is that it is a manifestation of impaired CO (Figure 12.5) and its significance is that it demonstrates the sequence of events that affect the cardiac chambers and result in impaired CO. Spontaneous inspiration

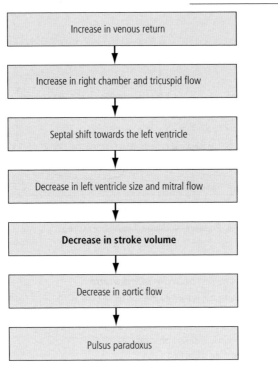

Figure 12.5 Pulsus paradoxus

decreases pericardial pressure (secondary to negative intrathoracic pressure). Note that during positive pressure ventilation, the lowest intrathoracic pressure occurs during expiration.

Echocardiographic features of acute tamponade
Two-dimensional features
- Mandatory presence of a pericardial effusion and, if large enough, the appearance of a 'swinging' heart. This is the echocardiography starting point; therefore, if there is not an effusion on 2D—revise your tamponade diagnosis. Look for something else to explain the haemodynamic changes.

- Cardiac chamber collapse (Figure 12.6). It is important to note that the thin-walled cardiac chambers (RA then RV) are the

(a)

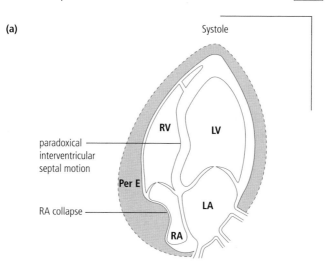

(b)

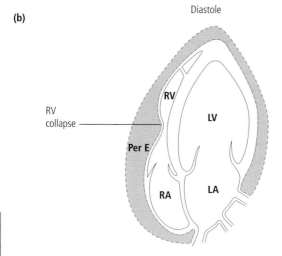

Figure 12.6 Right-sided chamber collapse in tamponade. (a) RA systolic collapse with paradoxical septal motion (with respiration). (b) RV diastolic collapse. Per E: pericardial effusion

first to be affected by the elevated pericardial pressures. The exception to this rule is the LA, which, although thin walled, is tethered to the pulmonary veins so will rarely collapse. RA systolic collapse is an early sign, followed by RV diastolic collapse, but may not occur in the presence of high PA pressures.

- Decrease in the size of the right chambers.
- Variation in size of RV and LV with respiration, which corresponds to pulsus paradoxus. During spontaneous respiration there is an increase in the size of the RV and a decrease in the size of the LV with inspiration, and with expiration the RV reduces and the LV increases in size. During positive pressure ventilation, the reverse will occur.
- Dilated IVC without partial collapse during spontaneous inspiration (sensitive but non-specific indicator).

Doppler features: Doppler is used to interrogate transvalvular flow patterns.

In spontaneous respiration, the RA inflow increases during inspiration, which will be reflected by an increased tricuspid valve E velocity. The opposite occurs with LA flow where an increase in flow occurs during expiration (increased mitral E velocity). Therefore, during inspiration, respiratory changes normally should be less than 20% by peak E velocity.

In the presence of a tamponade, these changes in transvalvular flow are exaggerated. Therefore, during inspiration the trans-tricuspid E wave velocity is increased by more than 40%, and the trans-mitral E wave velocity decreases by more than 25% (Figure 12.7). During positive pressure ventilation, the opposite is likely to occur.

A summary of the findings for pericardial tamponade is presented in Table 12.1 and a case example is provided on the CD.

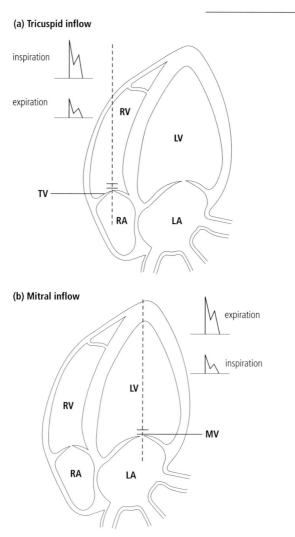

Figure 12.7 (a) Right and (b) left diastolic inflow in tamponade. PW Doppler sample gate placement is at the level of the atrioventricular valve leaflet tips. Note: Doppler waveforms will be inverted on TOE

Table 12.1 Clinical and 2D and Doppler echocardiographic features of pericardial tamponade

Clinical findings	2D echocardiography	Doppler
Low CO	Pericardial effusion	≥40% respiratory variation on TV valve inflow Doppler
Pulsus paradoxus	RA systolic collapse	≥25% respiratory variation on MV Doppler
Elevated jugular venous pressure	RV diastolic collapse Reciprocal RV and LV volume changes with respiration Dilated IVC	

Limitations in diagnosing pericardial pathology

- Aetiology of an effusion is not usually apparent on echocardiography.
- With a pericardial effusion secondary to myocardial rupture, the point of rupture is rarely identifiable.
- Beware the loculated pericardial effusion, particularly in the region of the atria, which may mimic a normal cardiac chamber.
- It may be difficult to identify pericardial thickening.
- Constrictive pericarditis is a topic in its own right but (1) the echocardiography features, especially the Doppler pattern with exaggerated respiratory variation, is very similar to the Doppler pattern seen in tamponade; (2) in the presence of these features and in the absence of a pericardial effusion, consider constrictive pericarditis; and (3) the case for this diagnosis is strengthened by the presence of a thickened pericardium (difficult to discern by echocardiography). Thickening of the pericardium may be better visualised on MRI.

Chapter 13

Ultrasound-guided regional anaesthesia

Paul Soeding

Learning objectives

1. Understand the anatomy relevant to regional anaesthesia.
2. Understand the current techniques of regional anaesthesia.
3. Describe the ultrasonographic anatomy of common nerve blocks.
4. Understand the technique of US-guided regional anaesthesia.
5. Describe the clinical benefits of US-guided regional anaesthesia.

Development of ultrasound-guided regional anaesthesia

In recent years there has been a renewed interest in the use of ultrasound (US) in regional anaesthesia. Since the first report of supraclavicular brachial plexus block using Doppler ultrasound by la Grange et al. in 1978, US-assisted nerve block has been described for localisation of the brachial and lumbar plexuses, and the sciatic and femoral nerves. A number of studies have shown US-guided techniques to have greater accuracy, quicker onset and less morbidity than conventional techniques.

An accurate knowledge of the nerves, their pathways and their relationship to vascular and anatomical structures is a prerequisite for successful regional anaesthesia. Surface anatomical landmarks can define the point of percutaneous injection, but once the needle passes through the skin it is directed unseen towards the target nerve. Often it is experience, together with various end-points such as loss of resistance or paraesthesia, that determine when the needle tip has reached its target.

Neurostimulation helps guide needle placement by activating nerves with a repetitive stimulating current from the needle tip. When the tip is in close proximity to the nerve, a motor or sensory response is elicited. As with all landmark techniques, neurostimulation essentially remains a blind technique. The risk of needle contact with vascular and neural structures remains, and in some patients, despite an elicited motor response, there is inexplicable failure of anaesthesia. Mechanical contact with nerves, intraneural injection or local anaesthetic toxicity can all result in neuropraxia. If nerve contact and vascular puncture can be avoided, morbidity is likely to be reduced. The complications common to all regional anaesthesia are failure, intravenous injection and neuropraxia.

Ultrasonography of nerves

Transducers

Modern US transducers comprise an array of piezoelectric elements that transmit and receive the sound waves. As the sound waves travel through tissue they are reflected at interfaces of altered acoustic impedance and it is these reflected waves that form a real-time sonographic image of the neural anatomy. Linear array transducers have multiple channels that emit parallel beams for enhancement of resolution, whereas sector transducers with divergent beams provide less resolution. The wavelength of transmission determines penetration depth, with smaller wavelengths having less tissue penetration, but higher image resolution. As frequency decreases, tissue penetration is increased but image resolution is diminished. Transducers with a frequency range between 5 and 15 MHz enable greater flexibility when examining different anatomical regions for neural elements.

Modern US systems enable high-resolution imaging of nerves by using appropriate software to enhance tissue contrast. Subcutaneous tissues reflect sound waves at varying degrees, depending on acoustic impedance. The manner in which the dynamic range of this input signal is processed determines the image quality on screen. High-level grey-scale contrast results in a precisely defined sonographic image.

Sonographic appearance of nerves

The appearance of a peripheral nerve depends on its size and the angle of insonation. Connective tissue surrounding nerve fascicles is often strongly reflected, producing a bright (hyperechoic) circular or oval rim on transverse scanning. The interior of the nerve, however, appears dark (hypoechoic) and can have a granular appearance. In the long axis, nerves appear as a band of strongly reflective, interrupted parallel lines, distinguished from tendons which have a continuous linear pattern. The linear fascicular pattern is a feature of larger nerves and is absent in small nerves.

The sonographic appearance of neural structures may be altered if the angle of insonation is oblique, and reflection is returned tangentially to the transducer (Figure 13.1). In such situations nerve rims

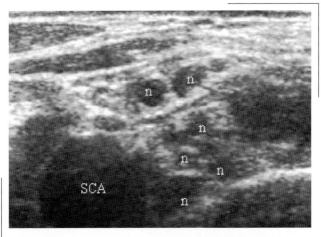

Figure 13.1 Supraclavicular sonogram of neural elements (n) adjacent to the subclavian artery (SCA)

may appear hypoechoic rather than hyperechoic in relation to surrounding tissues. This appearance due to oblique reflection is known as anisotrophy and is dependent on examination technique.

Surrounding vascular structures appear anechoic with pulsatile arterial vessels often identifiable. Veins are non-pulsatile and easily compressed by surface pressure. Fat and muscle (except perimysium) appear hypoechoic, tendons are hyperechoic, and bone is strongly hyperechoic.

Technique of US-guided regional anaesthesia

Ultrasound-guided regional anaesthesia has the same requirements of monitoring and resuscitation as any other regional technique. Initial preparation involves choosing the appropriate settings of frequency and gain and placing the probe in a sterile sheath or glove with ultrasonic gel for sterility. Removing the air from the injection syringe, tubing and regional needle is mandatory because injected air grossly obscures sonographic anatomy.

Ultrasound examination involves gentle pressure on the skin to avoid distortion, using fine movements of the probe to visualise the target nerves and surrounding anatomy (Figure 13.2). CFD can help

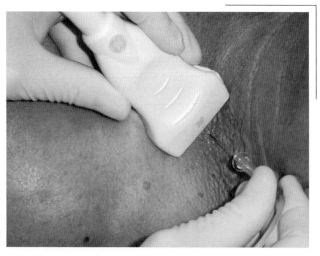

Figure 13.2 Regional anaesthesia using an ultrasound probe

identify vascular structures and gentle pressure can compress venous structures, thus distinguishing them from arterial vessels. Once the target nerve is identified sonographically, the image is centred and a direct route for needle advancement is chosen.

The probe is held either transversely or longitudinally and local infiltration is applied to the skin 1 cm from the probe. The needle is carefully advanced through the skin, only advancing it a few millimetres. The needle tip position is monitored on the screen and if not readily seen, can be identified by a gentle jiggling of the needle shaft, which causes adjacent tissue movement. The needle tip is advanced under direct vision, avoiding contact with vascular or neural structures. Once the tip is placed adjacent to the target nerve, the local anaesthetic solution is injected and monitored as it invests the nerve. For each target nerve the needle tip can be repositioned and local anaesthetic injected separately. Because the injection can be accurately placed, often less total volume is required. Placement of catheters is also facilitated by ultrasound imaging, ensuring the catheter lies adjacent to the nerve as it is advanced into place.

The brachial plexus

The brachial plexus originates from the cervical (C5–8) and thoracic (T1) nerve roots, which form the superior, middle and inferior trunks that travel down the posterior triangle of the neck into the supraclavicular region where they divide at the lateral edge of the first rib. These divisions pass infraclavicularly to form cords around the axillary artery before entering the axilla. The classic pattern shown in Figure 13.3 is an idealised configuration because anatomic variations do occur.

Ultrasonography of the interscalene region

The posterior triangle of the neck is bordered by the sternocleidomastoid muscle (SCM) anteriorly, the trapezius muscle posteriorly and the clavicle at the base. As shown in Figure 13.4, the interscalene groove (ISG) is palpable between the anterior and middle scalene muscles. At C6 it lies adjacent to the lateral edge of the SCM, or may be covered by this muscle. The external jugular vein (EJV) often lies superficially in this vicinity.

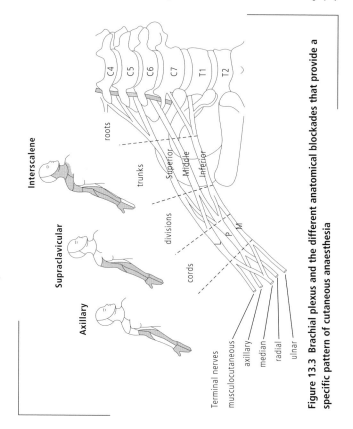

Figure 13.3 Brachial plexus and the different anatomical blockades that provide a specific pattern of cutaneous anaesthesia

Examination begins by placing the US probe on the neck, lateral to the cricoid cartilage, and slowly moving it laterally over the clavicular head of the SCM. Identification of the carotid artery, internal jugular vein (IJV) and adjacent thyroid tissue are reference landmarks for positioning the probe.

As the probe is positioned in the oblique sagittal plane, the ISG comes into view, identified by a characteristic double-hump appearance of the scalenus anterior (SA) and medius (SM) muscles. The muscles are separated by a fatty tissue space of 4–5 mm, which forms the interscalene space (ISS) and is an important anatomical compartment containing the plexus.

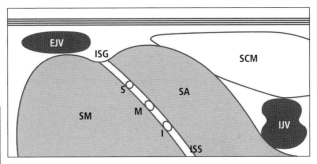

Figure 13.4 Sonographic anatomy of the brachial plexus in the interscalene region. S, M, I: superior, middle and inferior trunks

Within the ISS, the roots and/or trunks of the brachial plexus appear as hypodense nodules positioned against the anterior border of the SM. Deep and medial to these trunks, the acoustic shadow of the C6 transverse process may be seen. The vertebral artery and vein may also be identified anterior to this bony process with nerve roots posterior to the vertebral vessels.

Ultrasonography of the supraclavicular region

The transducer is placed above the mid-point of the clavicle (C) or, alternatively, may be directed caudally from the interscalene region, following the imaged brachial plexus downwards and laterally to reach the supraclavicular region. The key structure for orientation is the subclavian artery (SCA) located between the scalene muscles. CFD can be used to identify this vessel, as well as distinguish neural elements from arterial and venous branches (in particular, supra-scapular and transverse cervical branches).

In the supraclavicular fossa the superior, middle and inferior primary trunks divide into their anterior and posterior branches, which appear as a cluster of nodules located cephaloposterior to the subclavian artery (Figure 13.1). Distribution can vary, with elements of the inferior trunk, for example, sometimes positioned inferior to the artery, resulting in ulna-sparing during blockade.

The omohyoid muscle (OM) is seen superficially overlying the neural and vascular elements and the strong reflective signal of the first rib is noted inferiorly. The cervical pleura can be imaged

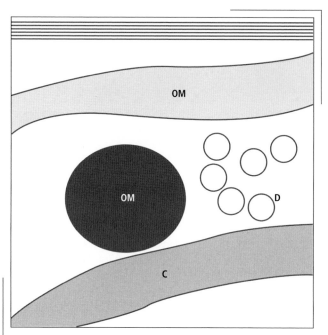

Figure 13.5 Sonographic anatomy of the brachial plexus in the supraclavicular region

medially behind the rib. As the needle tip is directed towards the plexus, medial angulation of the needle is visually directed to avoid inadvertent pleural puncture.

Ultrasonography of the infraclavicular region

As shown in Figure 13.6, for proximal infraclavicular techniques, the probe is placed below the midpoint of the clavicle overlying the pectoralis major. The plexus is located deep to the subclavian muscle and clavipectoral fascia, and itself lies on part of the serratus anterior. Often a lower US frequency is required for adequate penetration. Deep to these structures the ribs appear highly reflective and the pleura (Pl) is easily identified.

CFD is helpful for identifying the axillary artery (A) and also its thoracoacromial branch. More distal branches of the artery include

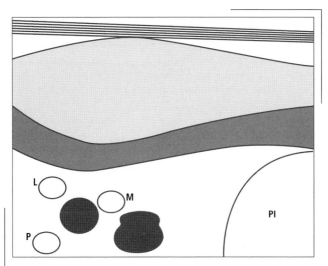

Figure 13.6 Sonographic anatomy of the brachial plexus in the infraclavicular region

the long thoracic, subscapular and humeral circumflex arteries. The axillary vein (V) is located medial to the artery and receives the cephalic vein at this level of the clavipectoral triangle.

The plexus divisions are initially located cranial to the axillary artery and as they travel over the first rib, they group together to form medial (M), lateral (L) and posterior (P) cords around the artery. The medial cord is often positioned between the artery and vein.

At the distal infraclavicular level the plexus lies deep to the pectoralis major (PM) and minor (Pm). The PM appears thick and overlies the Pm, with a strongly reflective hyperechoic perimysium separating the two muscles. The Pm tendon can be identified and followed laterally as it inserts onto the coracoid process. The neurovascular bundle can be found lying inferior and medial to this reference point.

Ultrasonography of the axillary region

The distribution of nerve position can vary as shown in Figure 13.7. There may be multiple venous structures present, which require identification before injection of local anaesthetic.

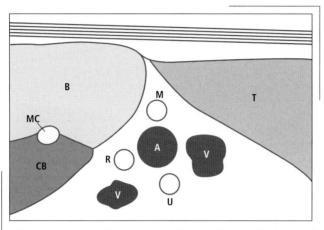

Figure 13.7 Sonographic anatomy of the brachial plexus in the axillary region

The axillary artery (A) enters the axilla and lies within the internal bicipital groove formed by the biceps (B) and coracobrachialis (CB) muscles superiorly, and the triceps (T) inferiorly.

A transverse view of the artery is obtained by placing the probe 90° over the sulcus, adjacent to the pectoral fold. The nerves are positioned around the artery and, in general, the median nerve (M) lies anterior, the ulna nerve (U) inferior and the radial nerve (R) posterior to the artery. The musculocutaneous nerve (MC) originates high in the axilla and travels within the body of the CB, which accounts for its sparing during axillary brachial plexus anaesthesia.

The lumbosacral plexus

The lumbar plexus (T12, L1–4) is located deep within the psoas muscle and lies anterior to the transverse processes of each lumbar vertebra. The sacral plexus (L3–4, S1–4) passes through the greater and lesser sciatic foramina. The lumbosacral plexus supplies the motor and sensory innervation of the leg, predominately via the femoral nerve anteriorly and the sciatic nerve posteriorly.

Ultrasonography of the femoral nerve

The femoral nerve (L2–4) is the largest branch of the lumbar plexus and passes beneath the inguinal ligament in a groove between the psoas and iliacus (Ili) muscles. It is both a sensory and a motor nerve, with blockade producing sensory anaesthesia of the upper leg anteriorly and the medial calf, and an inability to abduct the leg or extend the lower leg. It lies immediately lateral to the femoral artery (A) and is covered by the fascia lata (Fl) and fascia iliaca (Fi) (Figure 13.8). Because the nerve (N) is relatively superficial, a high-frequency probe placed just distal to the inguinal ligament will readily identify it and the spread of solution can be monitored for distribution beneath the fascial membrane.

The femoral nerve may be blocked in isolation, or in conjunction with the obtuator and lateral cutaneous nerves (3-in-1 block) when larger injection volumes spread perivascularly to reach the proximal lumbar plexus.

Ultrasonography of the sciatic nerve

The sciatic nerve (L3,4, S1–3; Figure 13.9) exits the pelvis through the greater sciatic foramen to enter the leg between the greater trochanter (GT) and ischial tuberosity (IT). It is a large nerve located deep to the

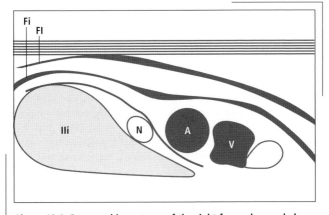

Figure 13.8 Sonographic anatomy of the right femoral nerve below the inguinal ligament

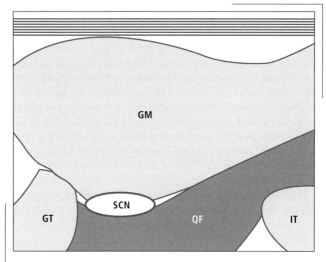

Figure 13.9 Sonographic anatomy of the sciatic nerve in the infragluteal region. QF: quadratus femoris

gluteus maximus (GM) and medius muscles, and therefore requires examination using a lower frequency probe. In a small percentage of patients the sciatic nerve (SCN) may have a high bifurcation, dividing it into tibial and peroneal branches as it emerges from the sciatic foramen. At this level the posterior femoral cutaneous nerve also emerges.

Blockade of the SCN will provide anaesthesia to the foot and lower extremity to distal to the knee. There are many classical approaches, with patients being positioned supine, lateral or semi-prone. The midpoint between the GT and IT, the posterior superior iliac crest, the sacral hiatus, GM and the midpoint of the thigh have all been used as landmarks to guide needle puncture for regional anaesthesia. Complications include failure, haematoma and intra-neural injection.

Ultrasound can be used to scan the thigh posteriorly and identify the SCN as it travels down to the popliteal fossa. It is most superficial in the subgluteal region and suitable for blockade at this point. Imaging can be difficult if the beam is not perpendicular to the nerve and thus poor muscle penetration occurs. Imaging in the popliteal fossa also identifies the nerve, the point at which it divides and the relationship between the peroneal and tibial nerves.

Specific regional blocks

Psoas compartment block: The lumbar plexus has sensory innervation of the lower limb from the thigh to the medial malleolus, the anterior upper leg and the lower abdomen. The psoas compartment block attempts to block the nerve roots as they emerge from the intervertebral foramina. The plexus lies within a fascial compartment between the quadratus lumborum and psoas muscles. Many approaches are described, often using the L3,4 vertebral bodies as reference points for needle insertion. Imaging of the plexus with US has been described, but can be difficult because it is a deep structure and adjacent to the vertebral column.

Epidural anaesthesia: In adults, US imaging of the epidural space is poor, even with a low-frequency probe. The epidural space is deeply situated and surrounded by the bony vertebral column. Ultrasound has been used to identify vertebral landmarks in obesely gravid patients and reduce the number of attempts of puncture for epidural catheter placement. In infants and children, however, the incomplete ossification of vertebra enables US to accurately visualise the epidural space, puncture of the ligamentum flavum and catheter placement.

Peripheral nerves

Many of the peripheral nerves around the elbow, knee, wrist and ankle are superficial structures that are identifiable on US examination, which is performed as described above.

Chapter 14

Ultrasound-guided vascular access

Colin Royse

Learning objectives

1. Understand the ultrasound equipment required for vessel cannulation.
2. Understand the basic techniques of US-guided vascular access.
3. Understand how to measure flow in small vessels.
4. Describe examples of vessel cannulation.

Development of ultrasound-guided vascular access

Anaesthetists, intensive care physicians and other perioperative medicine specialists have traditionally used blind techniques to cannulate peripheral vessels such as the internal jugular vein (IJV) or femoral artery (FA). Successful cannulation relies on knowledge of surface anatomy, experience, and an expectation that the patient's anatomy will be typical. Although an experienced operator will be successful in most instances, there is an incidence of failure and complications related to incorrect positioning of the needle during cannulation and, occasionally, catastrophic disasters occur. Patients do not always 'follow the rules'! Most problems arise as a result of the anatomy varying from the usual. It is not possible even for an experienced operator to perform a procedure accurately if the anatomy is aberrant. The path of the needle may also deflect the structures, especially the more rigid arteries, or for compressible structures such as veins, the needle may transfix the vessel. The concept of US-guided vascular access is very simple: identification of anatomy with ultrasound increases the likelihood of successful cannulation of vessels and reduces the risk of complications related to multiple needle passes or aberrant anatomy. Insertion of the needle under direct guidance will improve accuracy. Probe types and the techniques for imaging the vessels most commonly cannulated in perioperative medicine will be discussed.

Equipment requirements

The types of transducer (linear- or phased-array) have been described in previous chapters. For vessel cannulation, a linear-array transducer is a better choice than a phased-array type; however, if the only transducer available is a cardiac phased-array, it can still be useful for the cannulation of large vessels. A linear-array transducer can be used to measure flow with Doppler in parallel vessels and assumes an insonation angle of 60°. It is very difficult and inaccurate to attempt to measure flow in a parallel vessel with a phased-array cardiac transducer.

The second consideration is to choose the highest frequency transducer that will provide imaging for the depth of vessel that is to be cannulated. For most vessels, the best images are obtained using high-frequency transducers (e.g. 10–15 MHz). However, such transducers are limited to a depth of approximately 4 cm for good imaging. In cases such as accessing the FA in an obese patient, the vessel may not be easily seen and a lower frequency transducer may provide better imaging, although the resolution will be poorer, but for a large vessel such as the FA, the problem of high fidelity resolution is less critical.

Obtaining the best image
1. Select the most appropriate transducer.
2. Position yourself so that your eye, the needle, the vessel to be cannulated and the machine are in a straight line. It is easiest if you do not have to turn your head to see the images.
3. Have ultrasound gel and a marking pen at hand.

4. Be generous when applying the gel, but do not apply it near where the marker pen will be used.

5. Optimise the machine gain and depth settings. For most vessels a depth of 3–5 cm is ideal because it will project the vessel as a large image (make the vessel fill ≈two-thirds of the screen). Increase the gain so that the image appears brighter than necessary. These settings are particularly important when imaging a vessel while working at a distance from the screen.

6. First, apply light pressure because it will soon be apparent that veins are very compressible and the structure that needs to be imaged may be inadvertently obscured.

7. If a Doppler examination is to be performed, locate the vessel in transverse section first and then rotate the probe to image in the longitudinal section. This is particularly important when imaging small vessels, such as the radial artery, that are difficult to find in the longitudinal section.

8. In the beginner stages of vessel imaging, it is easier to find the vessel using ultrasound and mark its location (the 'find and mark' technique), and then perform the procedure without using ultrasound, because it will be quicker than by direct vision.

9. With experience, the procedure will be performed under direct vision, so the probe must be in a sterile sheath and held by one hand and the needle inserted with the other. This becomes easier with practice.

10. A full-sized echocardiography machine is not necessary to image vessels. Small portable point-of-care ultrasound machines are available with linear-array transducers (Figure 14.1) and their advantage is that they can be placed closer to the operator performing the procedure.

Cannulation techniques

The find-and-mark technique

In the find-and-mark technique, the vessel is located with ultrasound and its direction marked on the skin surface. Note the depth of the vessel from the skin surface. Vessel cannulation is performed in the usual manner. This is a very quick technique to execute and does

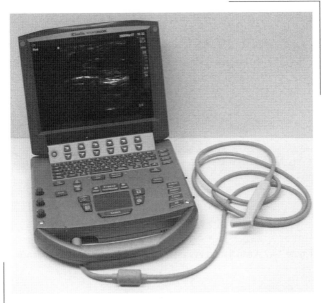

Figure 14.1 The Sonosite MicroMaxx is a point-of-care ultrasound machine that is fully cardiac capable, as well as being suitable for surface examinations

not require the additional expertise of holding the probe and inserting a needle at the same time.

Hold the probe in one hand and the marking pen in the other. Move the probe in transverse section to centre the vessel in the middle of the screen, which corresponds to the vessel overlying the middle of the transducer. Mark distally and proximally so that the direction of the vessel is clearly outlined. Note where the vessel diameter is largest and place a mark in the transverse plane. Finally, note the depth of the vessel and its relationship to other structures.

Direct vision
The technique of direct US-guided cannulation will develop with experience. The probe must be in a sterile sheath and held by one hand and the needle inserted with the other (Figure 14.2). This technique is

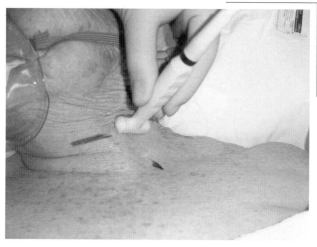

Figure 14.2 Cannulating vessels with real-time ultrasound guidance

definitely more difficult to do initially, but once the operator is confident with both holding the probe over the site that needs to be cannulated and then cannulating while looking at the screen rather than at the skin, it is certainly a more accurate method. The needle is not shown on the image as a needle, but as a point of ultrasound dropout that indents the tissues as it passes through them. This is the most difficult aspect of the technique, but 'jiggling' the needle slightly as it is advanced will assist in showing the tissues indenting at the point of the needle. Generally, the depth and direction of the needle is followed, which allows the operator to change the angle of the needle as it approaches the vessel. Veins are very compressible and the needle will commonly indent the vein before it punctures it. In fact, the vein 'impales' itself on the needle rather than the needle puncturing the vein. If the needle is passed too rapidly, it may transfix the vein.

Once the operator is confident with the procedure, there is no doubt that there will be more success with cannulating difficult vessels using this technique than with the find-and-mark technique.

Cannulation of specific vessels

Internal jugular vein

When imaging the internal jugular vein (IJV) with ultrasound, the middle portion of the vessel is shown lying anterior and lateral to the carotid artery, and may completely overlie the carotid artery proximally or distally (Figure 14.3). The extent to which the vein overlies the artery is very variable, which makes it quite easy to cannulate the artery by mistake, and the vein is very easy to compress with light pressure (Figure 14.4). For me, these were two difficulties to overcome when using ultrasound guidance. I was taught as a registrar to place the needle on the medial aspect of sternocleidomastoid muscle and aim laterally (towards the ipsilateral nipple), placing my fingers over the carotid artery to 'move it away from the vein', but the IJV usually lies lateral to the sternocleidomastoid muscle and is usually largest at the level of the cricothyroid cartilage. I also noticed that when palpating the carotid artery, the IJV was completely squashed. Accordingly, my cannulation technique has now changed to inserting the needle at the level of the cricoid cartilage lateral to the sternocleidomastoid muscle, and not pressing on the neck at all during needle insertion.

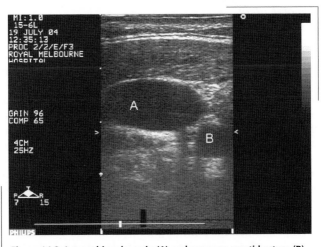

Figure 14.3 Internal jugular vein (A) and common carotid artery (B) on ultrasound image

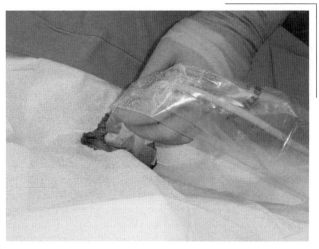

Figure 14.4 Philips 15-MHz linear-array probe is placed in a sterile sheath and positioned over the internal jugular vein

Femoral artery

Traditionally, the relationship between the femoral vein, artery and nerve is learnt at medical school as 'NAVYVAN'; that is, Nerve, Artery and Vein on the patient's right and Vein, Artery and Nerve proceeding laterally on the patient's left. These structures are easily identified with ultrasound and it soon becomes apparent that their location and orientation are not always as consistent with what has been taught (Figure 14.5). The major difference between the neck and the groin is the depth at which the blood vessels exist, particularly in obese patients. It is easiest to locate the structures by placing the probe in the transverse plane. Whereas the IJV is usually 1–2 cm deep, the femoral artery and vein are 2–4 cm, and in obese patients the depth settings may need to be increased to 5 cm or more. Furthermore, the vein does not always lie next to the artery, but may overlap it, superficially or deeply.

The find-and-mark method is generally sufficient for cannulation of the femoral vessels, but if they are very deep the US-guided technique will have to be used. One problem with femoral vein cannulation is that if the operator inadvertently strikes the femoral artery,

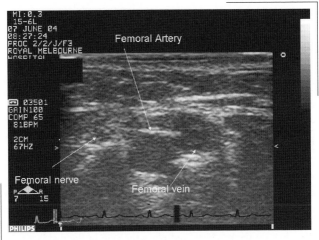

Figure 14.5 Location of the femoral nerve, artery and vein on ultrasound image

a haematoma will rapidly form and compress the vein making it very difficult, if not impossible, to successfully cannulate it. Imaging the area with ultrasound will usually show that the vein is compressed.

Radial artery

Why it is sometimes difficult to cannulate the radial artery even when a very good pulse can be felt? The problem is more noticeable for small arteries such as the radial or brachial. Insertion of the needle can displace the vessel and therefore the needle glances over it rather than punctures it. This problem is accentuated if there is a fascial plane lying between the skin and the vessel that is to be cannulated, which is certainly the case when cannulating the radial artery. It is a useful exercise to practise 'hand–eye' coordination by cannulating small vessels, such as the radial artery, under ultrasound guidance. If you can cannulate a small vessel, then you can cannulate any vessel! You will also appreciate the difficulty of the vessel moving as the needle approaches it, and thus start using the technique whereby you sit the needle tip on top of the vessel and then rapidly perform the final puncture to avoid displacement.

PICC line insertion

Typically, PICC line insertion has been the domain of either the anaes-thetist or the radiologist. Anaesthetists cannulate the vein as they would cannulate any other vein, whereas radiologists tend to use ultrasound to directly image the vessel as they insert the needle. If a vein is easily seen in the antecubital fossa, then one could argue that ultrasound is not necessary, but in many cases PICC lines are inserted after patients have had multiple peripheral venous catheters and it may be difficult or impossible to see or palpate the veins. The basic technique of US-guided cannulation is as has been described; that is, find-and-mark or using direct vision. Either technique is useful when a catheter is being placed in the veins proximal to the antecubital fossa because they are often deeper under the skin than in the forearm. The trick is to use very light pressure and plenty of gel; even slight pressure can compress the vessel. Set the depth to 1–2 cm, depending on the machine, and place the vein in the middle of the screen, which corresponds to the middle of the transducer and will assist with needle insertion. Insert the needle slowly, watching the vein indent before it is punctured. Once the vein resumes its round shape after the needle has indented it, assume that the needle tip lies in the

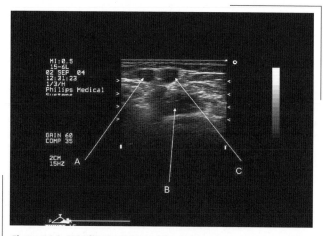

Figure 14.6 PICC line insertion. A, C: superficial veins at the level of the antecubital fossa; B: brachial artery

vein. At this stage, put down the transducer probe and aspirate on the needle to confirm placement. The rest of the PICC technique is usually performed with a Seldinger (using a guidewire) approach.

How to differentiate arteries from veins

There are three ways to help differentiate an artery from a vein.
1. Veins are easily compressed with light pressure whereas arteries are not.
2. Arteries are pulsatile whereas veins are not.
3. CFD will identify the vessel and determine the direction of flow (downstream or upstream). Remember the colour-coding convention: Blue is flow Away, Red is flow Towards the transducer (BART).

Chapter 15
Education and training

Colin Royse, Alistair Royse and Garry Donnan

> ## Learning objectives
> 1. Getting started in ultrasound
> 2. Further educational opportunities

Getting started in ultrasound

Originally, radiology was the only specialty to use ultrasound, but in the 1970s obstetricians and cardiologists started using it more frequently and subsequently specialists in paediatrics, anaesthetics, orthopaedics, and general and vascular surgery, in particular, have incorporated this technology into their practice with increasing enthusiasm.

One of the hurdles for new uses of ultrasound is the expectation by competitive craft groups that the level of knowledge must be equivalent to their established practice, even though the application of the technology may be different. This has the effect of impeding the development of ultrasound in the new area of application; for example, in anaesthesia, echocardiography was first introduced into cardiac surgery and cardiac anaesthetists were providing a diagnostic level of echocardiography in addition to using the technologies for intraoperative monitoring of cardiac function and haemodynamics. There were considerable internal and external pressures to only commence using this technology in a very advanced manner from the outset, but surprisingly ultrasound was taken up enthusiastically by cardiac anaesthetists because it was far more powerful than their existing invasive haemodynamic monitoring. The pressure exerted on them resulted in very rapid training in advanced echocardiography applications, but it also acted as a powerful disincentive for non-cardiac anaesthetists to develop an interest in ultrasound or echo-cardiography.

There are many uses of ultrasound and echocardiography in non-cardiac anaesthesia. Basic transthoracic imaging of the heart is the most useful assessment of haemodynamic volume resuscitation and in the hands of a skilled operator can provide much additional informa-tion. On a daily basis, surface ultrasound imaging of vessels for can-nulation for anaesthesia or surgery, placement of nerve blocks directly into nerve sheaths and imaging of the thyroid and trachea prior to percutaneous tracheotomy are just a few examples of the many prac-tical uses of ultrasound. These techniques are generally simple to learn and easy to implement. Most importantly, they can be incorporated into clinical practice before the study and experience necessary for advanced echocardiography is required. Indeed, using ultrasound for these purposes may never require the operator to have an advanced knowledge of echocardiography, yet will make a considerable positive impact on clinical practice. The concept that the technology is 'owned' by any specialty or group of individuals is fundamentally flawed. Ultrasound will be useful in some form to most specialties.

Two primary obstacles are encountered when wanting to start using ultrasound. The first is recognition, acceptance and desire that the technology be used in situations where previously it has not been. Resources are needed to purchase the equipment, but as the machines become more sophisticated, there are smaller and cheaper models that are more specifically focused for particular clinical applications. The second is formal training, which includes courses, diplomas or other theoretical educational activities, as well as practical experience. Both these obstacles can be overcome with an open mind, a strong desire, and determination.

When to seek further opinion

Do not be afraid to ask for a second opinion! There are many arti-facts and weird and wonderful anomalies that the average echo-cardiographer is unlikely to see. You may be performing a limited echocardiography examination and discover pathology that could affect the patient's future health (e.g. severe aortic stenosis). The echocardiography examination should be treated in the same manner as other diagnostic tests or medical practice, whereby appropriate referral to an expert in the area is arranged. In the case of identifying severe aortic stenosis, the anaesthetist may cancel the operation (e.g. hip replacement) and the patient be referred to a cardiologist for follow-up, which might lead to aortic valve replacement before the hip replacement can be safely performed.

Standards

The standards that you need to achieve in your practice of ultrasound are outlined in the guidelines and recommendations available on the American Society of Echocardiography website (http://asecho.org/ Guidelines_and_Documents/body_guidelines_and_documents.php# sca).

Further educational opportunities

Education for ultrasound in the perioperative environment has improved considerably in the past few years. There are textbooks on basic and advanced techniques, as well as short courses and work-shops run by organisations or societies. Until recently, there were not any educational opportunities other than institutional fellowships to provide the knowledge required to become an advanced diagnostic echocardiographer in the perioperative or critical care setting. The University of Melbourne now conducts short courses in point-of-care ultrasound and has developed a postgraduate diploma qualification in perioperative and critical care echocardiography (PGDipEcho), which is a very extensive course conducted entirely by distance education. The teaching is based on interactive tutorials with annotated images and video clips. Examination is also conducted via distance, so the knowledge can be obtained anywhere in the world. The web site is http://www.pharmacology.unimelb.edu.au/echocourse/faq.html. There are also two examinations for TTE, based in America or Europe, but these are not an education process.

References and further reading

References

American Society of Cardiovascular Anesthesiologists. Practice guidelines for perioperative transesophageal echocardiography: A report of the Task Force on Transesophageal Echocardiography. *Anesthesiology* 1996; 84: 986–1006.

Brunazzi MC, Chirillo F, Pasqualini M et al. Estimation of left ventricular diastolic pressures from precordial pulsed-Doppler analysis of pulmonary venous and mitral flow. *American Heart Journal* 1994; 128: 293–300.

Evangelista A, Gonzalez-Alujas MT. Echocardiography in infective endocarditis. *Heart* 2004: 90: 614–617.

Fox DJ, Khattar RS. Carcinoid heart disease: presentation, diagnosis, and management. *Heart* 2004; 90: 1224–1228.

Jacob S, Tong A. Role of echocardiography in the diagnosis and management of infective endocarditis. *Current Opinion in Cardiology* 2002; 17: 478–485.

Kallmeyer I, Collard C, Fox J et al. The safety of intraoperative transesophageal echocardiography: a case series of 7200 cardiac surgical patients. *Anaesthesia and Analgesia* 2001; 92: 1126–1130.

Kuecherer H, Muhiudeen I, Kusumoto F et al. Estimation of mean left atrial pressure from transesophageal pulsed Doppler echocardiography of pulmonary venous flow. *Circulation* 1990; 82: 1127–1139.

Kuhl HP, Hanrath P. The impact of transoesophageal echocardiography on daily clinical practice. *European Journal of Echocardiography* 2004; 5: 455–468.

Kusumoto F, Muhiudeen I, Keucherer H et al. Response of the inter-atrial septum to transatrial pressure gradients and its potential for predicting pulmonary capillary wedge pressure: an interoperative study using transesophageal echocardiography in patients during mechanical ventilation. *Journal of the American College of Cardiology* 1993; 21: 721–728.

la Grange P, Foster PA, Pretorius LK. Application of the Doppler ultrasound blood flow detector in supraclavicular brachial plexus block. *British Journal of Anaesthesia* 1978; 50: 965–967.

Milling TJ Jr, Rose J, Briggs WM et al. Randomized, controlled clinical trial of point-of-care limited ultrasonography assistance of central venous cannulation: The Third Sonography Outcomes Assessment Program (SOAP-3) Trial. *Critical Care Medicine* 2005; 33: 1764–1769.

Ranganathan N, Lam JH, Wigle ED, Silver MD. Morphology of the human mitral valve. II: The valve leaflets. *Circulation* 1970; 41: 459–467.

Royse CF, Barrington MJ, Royse AG. Transoesophageal echocardiography values for left ventricular end-diastolic area, pulmonary vein and mitral inflow Doppler velocities in patients undergoing coronary artery bypass surgery. *Journal of Cardiothoracic and Vascular Anesthesia* 2000; 14: 130–132.

Royse CF, Royse AG, Soeding PF, Blake DW. Shape and movement of the interatrial septum predicts change in pulmonary capillary wedge pressure. *Annals of Thoracic and Cardiovascular Surgery* 2001; 7: 79–83.

Vieillard-Baron A, Chergui K, Rabiller A et al. Superior vena caval collapsibility as a gauge of volume status in ventilated septic patients. *Intensive Care Medicine* 2004; 30: 1734–1739.

Yacoub MH, Cohn LH. Novel approaches to cardiac valve repair from structure to function: part II. *Circulation* 2004; 109: 1064–1072.

Further reading

Anderson B. *Echocardiography: The Normal Examination and Echocardiographic Measurements*. MGA Graphics, Queensland, 2002.

Angelsen B. *Ultrasound Imaging: Waves, Signals and Signal Processing*. Emantec, Norway, 2000.

Appelbe AF, Walker PG, Yeoh JK, Bonitatibus A, Yoganathan AP, Martin RP. Clinical significance and origin of artifacts in transesophageal echocardiography of the thoracic aorta. *Journal of the American College of Cardiology* 1993; 21: 754–760.

Auroy Y, Narchi P, Messiah A et al. Serious complications related to regional anaesthesia: results of a prospective survey in France. *Anesthesiology* 1997; 87: 479–486.

Bolotin G, Domany Y, de Perini L et al. Use of intraoperative epiaortic ultrasonography to delineate aortic atheroma. *Chest* 2005; 127: 60–65.

Cerqueira MD, Weissman NJ, Dilsizian V et al. American Heart Association Writing Group on Myocardial Segmentation and Registration for Cardiac Imaging. Standardised myocardial segmentation and nomenclature for tomographic imaging of the heart: a statement for healthcare professionals from the Cardiac Imaging Committee of the Council on Clinical Cardiology of the American Heart Association. *Circulation* 2002; 105: 539–542.

Cohen GI, White M, Sochowski RA et al. Reference values for normal adult transesophageal echocardiographic measurements. *Journal of the American Society of Echocardiography* 1995; 8: 221–230.

Cousins MJ, Bridenbaugh PO (eds). *Neural Blockade in Clinical Anaesthesia and Management of Pain*, 3rd edn. Lippincott Williams & Wilkins, Philadelphia, 1998.

Echo in Context program, Duke University School of Medicine website. Available at http://www.echoincontext.com

Evangelista A, Avegliano G, Elorz C et al. Transesophageal echocardiography in the diagnosis of acute aortic syndrome. *Journal of Cardiac Surgery* 2002; 17: 95–106.

Feigenbaum H, Armstrong WF, Ryan T. *Feigenbaum's Echocardiography*, 6th edn. Lippincott Williams & Wilkins, Philadelphia, 2005.

Gent R. *Applied Physics and Technology of Diagnostic Ultrasound*. Milner Publishing, South Australia, 1997.

Hartman GS, Yao FS, Bruefach M 3rd et al. Severity of aortic atheromatous disease diagnosed by transesophageal echocardiography predicts stroke and other outcomes associated with coronary artery surgery: a prospective study. *Anesthesia and Analgesia* 1996; 83: 701–708.

Marhofer P, Greher M, Kapral S. Ultrasound guidance in regional anaesthesia. *British Journal of Anaesthesia* 2005; 94: 7–17.

Neal JM, Hebl JR, Gerancher JC, Hogan QH. Brachial plexus anesthesia: essentials of our current understanding. *Regional Anesthesia and Pain Medicine* 2002; 27: 402–428.

Net Anatomy. Available at http://www.netanatomy.com/CSA/csa_frame.htm in the Thorax section.

Oka Y, Goldiner PLJ. *Transesophageal Echocardiography*. Lippincott Williams & Wilkins, Philadelphia, 1992.

Otto C. *Textbook of Clinical Echocardiography*. WB Saunders, Philadelphia, 2000.

Penco M, Paparoni S, Dagianti A et al. Usefulness of transesophageal echocardiography in the assessment of aortic dissection. *American Journal of Cardiology* 2000; 86: 53G–56G.

Rapp H, Folger A, Grau T. Ultrasound-guided epidural catheter insertion in children. *Anesthesia and Analgesia* 2005; 101: 333–339.

Rosenberger P, Shernan SK, Body SC, Eltzschig HK. Utility of intraoperative transesophageal echocardiography for diagnosis of pulmonary embolism. *Anesthesia and Analgesia* 2004; 99: 12–16.

Sidebotham D, Merry A, Leggett M. *Practical Perioperative Transesophageal Echocardiography.* Butterworth–Heinemann, Edinburgh, 2003.

Westmead Hospital Transoesophageal Echocardiographic Training Manual. Westmead Hospital, Sydney, 2003.

Glossary

2D two-dimensional

3D three-dimensional

A1 section of the anterior MV leaflet closest to the anterolateral commissure

A2 second (middle) section of the anterior MV leaflet

A3 section of the anterior MV leaflet closest to the posteromedial commissure

acoustic impedance resistance of a medium to the transmission of ultrasound; dependent on the density and compressibility of (and therefore, the speed of sound in) that medium; measured in rayl or 1 kg/m per s

acoustic shadowing failure of sound waves to pass a structure and all are reflected to the transducer, resulting in a dark area or shadow beyond the structure

acute aortic syndrome aortic disease that presents as acute chest pain

aliasing inaccurate representation of the Doppler shift being interrogated because a low sampling frequency is being used

ALMV anterior leaflet of the MV

ALPM anterolateral papillary muscle

ALTV anterior leaflet of the TV

anisotrophy effect of obliquely reflected sound waves on the resolution of the ultrasound image

anteflex flexing the probe tip anteriorly

AoR aortic root

aortic atheroma accumulation of lipid and cholesterol-containing plaque in the walls of the aorta (from the Greek 'athero' meaning gruel or paste)

aortic dissection tear originating in the intima of the aorta, resulting in abnormal blood flow, which may extend between the intimal and medial layers of the vessel and create a false lumen

Ap2ch apical 2-chamber view

Ap4ch apical 4-chamber view

artifact image that does not make physiological or anatomical sense

AV aortic valve

Bernoulli equation conservation of energy; relates the pressure drop along a tube to the velocity of the fluid in that tube, which enables conversion of velocity to pressure

blind spot   area of poor or absent imaging

BP   blood pressure

BSA   body surface area

CABG   coronary artery bypass grafting

cardiac mass   abnormal structure within a heart cavity or immediately adjacent to the heart

CFD   colour flow Doppler

CFM   colour flow mapping

CO   cardiac output

continuity principle   conservation of mass (i.e. provided nothing is added to or removed from a system, 'what goes in, must come out')

contrast resolution   see resolution

CS   coronary sinus

CVP   central venous pressure

CW   continuous wave

deceleration time (DT)   time taken for the E velocity to fall from peak to zero velocity (baseline) and reflects the time required for the left ventricular and atrial pressures to equalise in early diastole

Doppler effect   change in the frequency of a wave because of the relative velocity of the transmitter to the receiver

Doppler shift   difference between the transmitted and received frequencies

ECG   electrocardiogram

echodense   area appears white because of the high reflection of sound waves by highly reflective tissues or compounds (e.g. calcium, metal)

ED   emergency department

EF   ejection fraction

epiaortic ultrasound   during cardiac surgery, a high-frequency ultrasound transducer is placed in a sterile bag and closely approximated to the aortic wall to give high-quality ultrasound image resolution of the vessel

FAC   fractional area change

far field   the part of the ultrasound image that is far from the transducer (see also near field)

FAST   focused assessment with sonography for trauma

forward rotation   axial rotation of the ultrasound from 0 degrees (horizontal plane) to 90 degrees (vertical plane)

frequency   number of oscillations (waves) per second, measured in hertz

frequency aliasing   measured Doppler frequency is ambiguous to that of the receiver

frequency resolution   see resolution

GI   gastrointestinal

haemodynamics   combination of factors that influence the global performance of the heart, including preload, ventricular function and ventricular filling pressures

HCM   hypertrophic cardiomyopathy

hyperdynamic systolic function   LV contracts more vigorously than normal

Hz   hertz; unit of measurement of frequency

IV   intravenous

IVC   inferior vena cava

jiggle   move the needle tip up and down to help identify where it is on the screen

LA   left atrium

LAA   left atrial appendage

LAD   left anterior descending (artery)

LAP   left atrial pressure

LAX   long-axis view

LCC   left coronary cusp

LV   left ventricle

LVOT   left ventricular outflow tract

M-mode   motion mode (1-dimensional echocardiography)

MO   mid-oesophageal

MR   mitral regurgitation

MRI   magnetic resonance imaging

MV   mitral valve

NCC   non-coronary cusp

near field   the part of the ultrasound image that is close to the transducer. 'Near' and 'far' are defined by the mathematical relationship between the wavelength of the ultrasound beam and the effective diameter ('acoustic aperture') of the transducer array

neuropraxia   neural injury leading to temporary loss of function, which may progress to dysthesia and chronic pain syndrome

neurostimulation   localisation of peripheral nerve using a low-intensity electrical current to elicit a motor response

Nyquist limit   maximum Doppler shift (and therefore calculated blood velocity), which can be derived accurately, beyond which aliasing occurs. Defined as half the pulse repetition frequency

operator   sonographer performing and reporting the study

P1   lateral scallop of the posterior MV leaflet

P2   middle scallop of the posterior MV leaflet

P3   medial scallop of the posterior MV leaflet

PA   pulmonary artery

paraesthesia   sharp or painful 'electric' sensation or sensation of 'pins and needles' down the arm, indicating needle contact with a nerve

PEEP   positive end-expiratory pressure

pericardial effusion   accumulation of more than 10 mL of fluid in the pericardial space

pericardium   two layer (outer parietal, inner visceral) envelope enclosing the heart

PICC   percutaneously inserted central catheter; thin catheters made of Silastic or other low-irritant material and designed for long-term use

PISA   proximal isovelocity surface area

pitfall   normal anatomical variant that may be mistaken for pathology

PLAX   parasternal long-axis

PLMV   posterior leaflet of the MV

PLTV   posterior leaflet of the TV

PMPM   posteromedial papillary muscle

PRF   pulse repetition frequency

pulmonary embolism   substance that has originated from a distant location within the circulation and obstructs the pulmonary artery or a branch of the pulmonary artery; most commonly a thrombus, but may also be tumour fragments, air or fat

PV   pulmonary valve

PW   pulse wave

RCA   right coronary artery

RCC   right coronary cusp

resolution   ability to distinguish between two items with similar properties: spatial resolution refers to items that are physically close; temporal resolution is the ability to identify events occurring at short time intervals; contrast resolution is the ability to distinguish between echoes of similar amplitude; frequency resolution (in Doppler ultrasound) is the ability to resolve velocities

retroflex   flexing the probe tip posteriorly

RV   right ventricle

RVOT   right ventricular outflow tract

RVSP   right ventricular systolic pressure

RWMA   regional wall motion abnormality: area of myocardium working at a different grade from the rest of the myocardium

SAM   systolic anterior motion of the anterior mitral valve leaflet, leading to dynamic outflow obstruction in HCM. It is caused by the Venturi effect of accelerated blood flow through the LVOT

SAX   short-axis view

SEC   spontaneous echo contrast or 'smoke'; occurs in areas of low velocity blood flow and has a distinct swirling appearance

spatial resolution   see resolution

SV   stroke volume

SVC   superior vena cava

tamponade   physiological changes caused by fluid in the pericardium compressing the heart; characterised by low cardiac output, elevated right heart pressures and haemodynamic compromise

TDI   tissue Doppler imaging

temporal resolution   see resolution

TG   transgastric

TOE   transoesophageal echocardiography

TR   tricuspid regurgitation

transducer   device that converts a physical property (i.e. pressure wave of an ultrasound echo) to a form that can subsequently be processed (e.g. electrical signal)

TTE   transthoracic echocardiography

TV   tricuspid valve

ulna sparing   lack of anaesthesia to the ulna side of the hand when using an interscalene approach, because the inferior trunk of the brachial plexus is positioned inferiorly beneath the artery, which may limit exposure to the injection

ultrasound   sound with a frequency greater than 20 000 Hz

VCR   videocassette recorder

VTI   velocity–time integral

wavelength   distance between two identical points of a pressure wave

Index

Tables and figures have not been indexed, but are accessible through references from the text.

2D imaging mode, 15, 24–5, 84
    transthoracic echocardiography, 66, 68

acute aortic syndrome, 161
anaesthesia, *see* ultrasound-guided regional anaesthesia
anatomy, 38–47, 165
aneurysms
    aortic, 125, 158, 160–1
    ventricular, 113
annular calcification, 48, 141
annular dilatation, 134, 139, 143
aorta, 156–7, 161–2
    atheroma, 162
    basic views, 55
    echocardiography 'blind spots', 48
    flow reversal in, 134
aortic aneurysm, 125, 158
    repair of, 160–1
aortic arch, 48
aortic coarctation, 162
aortic dilatations, 158
aortic dissection (AD), 158–61
    repair of, 160–1
aortic regurgitation, 134, 137
aortic stenosis, 131–4
    echocardiography, 132, 134
aortic valves, 133–7
    basic views, 54–5
    fibroelastomas, 127

apical aneurysms, 125
apical window, 66–8, 71, 91
area of valves, 88–90, 147
arteries, 43, 195, *see also* aorta
    cannulation techniques, 196–7
    differentiating from veins, 199
    pulmonary, 48, 157–8
artifacts, 30–1
atheroma, 162
atrium, *see also* left atrial pressure; left atrium; right atrial pressure
    atrial reversal, 122
    myxomas, 127
    variants (pitfalls), 31–2
axillary region, 185–6

B (brightness) imaging mode, 15, 24–5
base of the heart, 41–3
Bernoulli equation, 85–7
bileaflet valves, 151
biprosthetic valves, 152
bleeding, prosthetic valves and, 153
'blind spots' in echocardiography, 47–8
blockades, *see* ultrasound-guided regional anaesthesia
blood flow, *see* Doppler imaging; flow patterns
blood vessels, *see* arteries; valves; veins
brachial plexus, 179, 181–6

caged ball (Starr Edwards) valves,

151
calculations, 88–90
  distance, 76, 78
cannulation techniques, 192–4
  specific vessels, 195–9
carcinoid syndrome, 143
cardiac anatomy, 41–6
  echocardiography blind spots,
      47–8
  echocardiography 'slices', 44,
      46
  variations in, 46–7
cardiac chambers, 55–6, 172
cardiac ischaemia, *see* ischaemic
      heart disease
cardiac masses, 125–30
cardiac output, 88–90
cardiac sources of embolus, 125
cardiac surgery, 8, 162
cardiac tamponade, *see* pericardial
      tamponade
cardiac ultrasound, *see*
      echocardiography
cardiomyopathies, 113–16
carotid artery, 195
cerebral injury, postoperative, 162
chambers, 55–6, 172
chest anatomy, 38–41
cleaning and disinfection of
      probes, 50
colour flow Doppler (CFD), 79, 84
  transthoracic echocardiography,
      64, 66, 68–9
colour flow mapping (CFM),
      16–18, 68
compliance curves (pressure-
      volume), 169
congenital valve problems, 131,
      137
continuity equations, 147–8
continuity principle, 89

continuous wave (CW) Doppler
      imaging, 16, 78–9, 84
  hypertrophic cardiomyopathy,
      115
contraindications to
      echocardiography, 5
controls, *see* equipment
coronary arteries, 43
critical care practice, 1–8, *see also*
      emergency departments;
      intensive care units
cutaneous anaesthesia, brachial
      plexus and, 181–3

deceleration time (DT), 147
degenerative calcific stenosis, 131,
      137
diastolic function, 103–5, 118–24
dilated cardiomyopathy, 114
direct vision technique, 193–4
distance calculations, 76, 78
Doppler imaging, 73–83
  inflow patterns, 64, 68–9
  mode controls, 26–8
  modes, 15–18
  pericardial tamponade, 174
  pulmonary vein, 101–2
  standard examination, 84–7
  tissue, 123

Ebstein's anomaly, 144
echocardiography, 2–5, *see also*
      equipment
  'blind spots', 47–8
  great vessels, 156–63
  individual anatomical
      variations, 46–7
  risks and limitations, 4–5,
      18–19
  transoesophageal, 4–5, 49–62
  transthoracic, 4–5, 63–72

education in ultrasound, 200–2
electrical interference, 18
emboli, 125, 153
emergency departments, *see also* critical care practice
aortic dissection in, 159–60
empty (hypovolaemic) state, 103–4
end-diastolic area (EDA), 96–7
endocarditis, 154–5
environmental factors (room configuration), 29–30
epiaortic ultrasound, 158, 162
epidural anaesthesia, 189
equations in Doppler imaging, 88–90
distance, 76, 78
equipment, 11–12, 14
care of probes, 49–50
for ultrasound-guided vascular access, 191–2
instrument layout and settings, 21–9

FAST, 6
femoral artery, cannulation of, 196–7
femoral nerve, 187
fibroelastomas, 127
fibrous skeleton, 42
field depth, 18
filling pressure estimates, 97, 100–2
find-and-mark technique, 192–3
flow patterns, 75–6, 79, 118, 120, 122
pericardial tamponade, 174
focused assessment with sonography for trauma (FAST), 6
frequency aliasing, 78

global ventricular function, 110–12
glossary, 207–11
great vessels, problems with, 156–63, *see also* aorta; pulmonary artery

haemodynamic assessment, 93–105
basic states, 93–4, 102–5
value in patient management, 104–5
heart, *see* cardiac...; echocardiography
hepatic vein Doppler imaging, 144
hypertrophic cardiomyopathy, 115–16
hypovolaemic (empty) state, 103–4

image quality, 20–37
artifacts and pitfalls, 30–2
factors affecting, 20–1
imaging modes, 15–18
controls on instruments, 24–8
imaging transducers, 14, 75–6, 178–9
incident transducer angles, 75
infective endocarditis, 154–5
inflow patterns, *see* flow patterns
infraclavicular region, 184–5
instruments, *see* equipment
intensive care units, 7–8, *see also* critical care practice
interatrial septum, 97, 100–2
septal variants, 32
internal jugular vein, cannulation of, 195
interscalene region, 181–3
intraoperative uses of ultrasound, 8, 162–3

intravenous line insertion, 198–9
ischaemic cerebral injury,
        postoperative, 162
ischaemic heart disease, 112–13,
        116–17

jet length and area, 149–50, *see
        also* flow patterns
jugular vein, cannulation of, 195

keyboard controls, 21

leaflets, *see* valve leaflets
left atrial pressure (LAP), 100–2,
        120
    filling pressure estimates, 97
left atrium
    mitral regurgitation and, 141
    thrombi, 125
left ventricle
    assessment of function, 111
    'blind spots' in
        echocardiography, 47–8
    mitral regurgitation and, 141
    regional wall motion
        abnormalities, 116–17
    segments of, 44
    thrombi, 125
    volume estimates (preload), 95
limitations of echocardiography,
        5, 18–19
lumbosacral plexus, 186–9

M-mode echocardiography, 15,
        18, 26–8, 95
masses, cardiac, 125–30
mean pressure gradients, 86
mean velocity, 85–6
measurement controls, 28–9
mechanical valves, 151
mitral annular calcification, 137

mitral inflow patterns, 114, 118,
        120
mitral regurgitation, 113, 139,
        141–2
mitral stenosis, 137, 139
mitral valve area (MVA), 147
mitral valves, 137–42
    echocardiography 'blind spots',
        48
modes, *see* imaging modes
myocardial diseases
        (cardiomyopathies), 113–16
myocardial infarction, 112–13,
        116–17
myocardial ischaemia, 112–13,
        116–17
myxoma, 127, 137

needle insertion, *see* cannulation
        techniques
nerve bundles, ultrasonography
        of, 6–7
nerves, *see also* femoral nerve;
        sciatic nerve
    appearance of, 179–80
    peripheral, 189
    ultrasonography of, 178–81
Nyquist limits, 78–9, 148

operator factors in image quality,
        20
output, cardiac, 88–90

pannus ingrowth, 153
papillary fibroelastomas, 127
parasternal window, 64–6, 71, 91
paravalvular leaks, 153
patent ductus arteriosus, 162
patients
    factors affecting image quality,
        21

haemodynamic assessment, 104–5
 individual variations, 46–7
 positioning, 63–4
peak pressure gradients, 86
peak velocity, 79, 85
percutaneous tracheostomy, 7
pericardial effusion, 166–9
 in acute tamponade, 172
 views for interrogating, 167
pericardial tamponade, 169–76
 clinical features of, 171–2
 echocardiographic features of, 172–6
 transvalvular flow patterns, 174
pericardiocentesis, 8
pericarditis, 166
pericardium, 164–76
 anatomy, 165
 physiology, 165–6
perioperative practice, 1–8
peripheral nerves, 189
physics of ultrasound, 9–11
PISA, 148
pitfalls (variants), 31–2
pleura, 164–6
pleural effusions, 169
point-of-care ultrasound, 192
positioning the patient, 63–4
postoperative ischaemic cerebral injury, 162
preload, *see* volume estimates
pressure gradients, 86–7
 valvular stenosis, 147
pressure half-time (PHT), 147
pressure-volume (compliance) curve, 169
probes
 basic manoeuvres, 51, 53
 care of, 49–50
prosthetic valves, 150–3

echocardiography 'blind spots', 48
proximal isovelocity surface area (PISA), 148
psoas compartment block, 189
pulmonary artery, 157–8
 echocardiography 'blind spots', 48
pulmonary embolism, 163
pulmonary regurgitation, 145
pulmonary stenosis, 145
pulmonary valves, 145–6
pulmonary vein Doppler, 101–2
pulmonary venous inflow pattern, 120, 122
pulse repetition frequency (PRF), 78
pulse wave (PW) Doppler imaging, 16, 76, 84
pulsus paradoxus, 171

radial artery, cannulation of, 197
red cells in blood vessels, 75–6
regional anaesthesia, *see* ultrasound-guided regional anaesthesia
regional wall motion abnormalities (RWMAs), 116–17
regurgitation, 134, 139–45, 149–50
report writing, 72
restrictive cardiomyopathy, 114
rheumatic fever, 132, 137, 143
right atrial pressure (RAP), 88
right ventricle
 assessment of function, 112
 assumptions in, 85
 failure, 104–5
right ventricular systolic pressure (RVSP), 87

risks of echocardiography, 4
room configuration, 29–30

sacral plexus, 186–9
sciatic nerve, 187–9
sector rotation, 51
septa, *see* interatrial septum
signal aliasing, 78, 84
Simpson's method, 95–6
single tilting disc (Bjork Shiley)
    valves, 151
sound, physics of, 8–11
spectral displays, 75, 84
standards for ultrasound, 202
stenosis, *see* valvular stenosis
stomach, transgastric views, 56–8
storage of probes, 49–50
subaortic stenosis, 132
subcostal window, 68–9, 71
subvalvular attachments, 142
supraclavicular region, 179,
    183–4
suprasternal window, 69, 71
surgery, 8, 162–3
systolic failure, 103, 105
systolic function estimates, 97

tamponade physiology, 169–76
thoracentesis, 8
thoracic anatomy, 38–41
thoracic aorta, 156–7
    diameters, 158
thrombi, 125, 153
tissue Doppler imaging (TDI), 123
tracheostomy, 7
trackball controls, 28–9
training in ultrasound, 200–2
transducers, 14, 75–6, 178–9
transoesophageal
    echocardiography (TOE), 3,
    49–62

4-step haemodynamic
    assessment, 104
basic manoeuvres, 51, 53
basic views, 53–8
care of probes, 49–50
risks and limitations, 4–5
standard examination, 50–8
'street map', 53–8
views for interrogating
    pericardial effusions, 167
vs. transthoracic, 4–5
transthoracic echocardiography
    (TTE), 3–4, 63–72, 89, 167
4-step haemodynamic
    assessment, 104
risks and limitations, 4–5
standard examination, 69–72
suggested order, 71
transducers, 14
vs. transoesophageal, 4–5
traumatic aortic disruption, 161
tricuspid regurgitation, 143–5
tricuspid stenosis, 143
tricuspid valves, 143–5
tumours (cardiac masses), 125–30

ultrasound, 1–8, 20–37
blood flow, *see* Doppler
    imaging; flow patterns
education and training, 200–2
heart, *see* echocardiography
machines, *see* equipment
nerves, 178–81
physics of, 9–11
system assumptions, 31
ultrasound-guided regional
    anaesthesia, 177–89
development of, 177–8
technique, 180–1
ultrasound-guided vascular access,
    190–9

development of, 190–1
obtaining the best images, 191–2
urinary retention, 8

valve leaflets, 141, 143
    aortic regurgitation and, 134
    bileaflet valves, 151
    coaptation, 134, 141–2
    mitral regurgitation and, 139
valves, *see also* aortic valves;
        mitral valves
    anatomy, 41–3
    area of, 88–90, 147
    problems with, 131–55
    prosthetic, 150–3
    variants (pitfalls), 32
valvular regurgitation, 134,
        139–45, 149–50
valvular stenosis
    aortic, 131–4
    evaluation of, 147–8
    mitral, 137–9
    prosthetic valves, 153
    pulmonary, 145
    tricuspid, 143

vascular access, ultrasound-
        guided, 190–9
vascular structures, imaging of, 6
vasodilation, 105
vegetations (cardiac masses),
        125–30
veins
    cannulation techniques, 195
    differentiating from arteries,
        199
    pulmonary, 101–2
velocity, 75–6, 85–7
ventricles, 44, *see also* left
        ventricle; right ventricle
    aneurysms, 113
    global function, 110–12
    problems with, 110–30
    septal defects, 113
    variants (pitfalls), 32
volume estimates (preload), 95–7

wall thickening, 116–17
websites, 202
windows, for TTE, 64–9
writing reports, 72

Instructions

This mini-CD product will operate on PC or Mac. If you have a PC the program will launch automatically once inserted into your CD-ROM drive. If it does not launch, open your file manager and double click the MGH.EXE file. If you have a Mac, load the CD-ROM then click on the icon that matches your operating system (Classic or OSX).

Minimum system requirements

- Operating system: Win 2000, Win XP and Win 2003, Mac Classic 9.2, OSX 10.26 or greater.
- CD-ROM drive or DVD drive
- Monitor resolution 800 × 600 or higher @ thousands of colours